WHAT ABOUT MY CALCIUM?

A COMPLETE PLANT BASED GUIDE FOR CALCIUM HEALTH

We may not want to live longer, but we certainly desire to live healthy!

Comics: **Ramnath Patil** | Editor: **Nandita Kapadia**

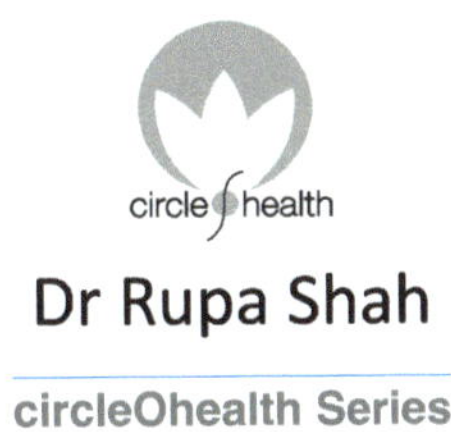

Dr Rupa Shah

circleOhealth Series

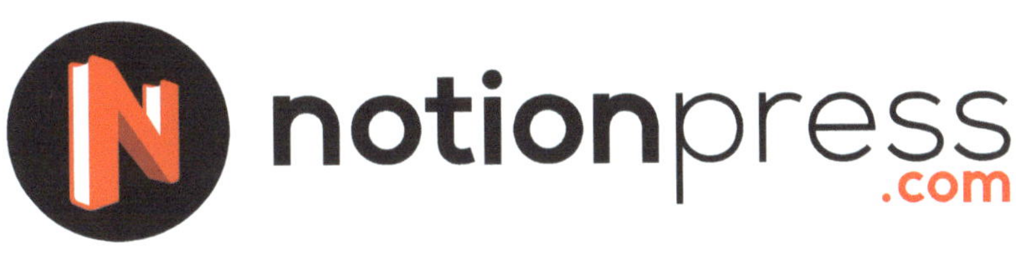

INDIA • SINGAPORE • MALAYSIA

ISBN 979-8-89066-764-9

Mobile No. +91-9821248428
www.healthrevolution.in
e-mail: drupashah@gmail.com

Dedication

This book is dedicated to my husband Dr Atul K Shah who has been my best critic, advisor and supporter in my journey towards wellness.

Acknowledgment

This book would not have been completed without the following people whose support is deeply appreciated:

I would like to thank my team members (in alphabetical order): Mahesh Jadhav, Manju Parval, Neha Doshi, Ruchika Chitrabhanu and Saroj Choudhury.

My heartfelt thanks to Shri Varidhibhai Thakkar, Richa Hingle, Jinal Rathod, and Parul Mehta for sharing their recipes for this book.

My deepest gratitude to Dr John McDougall, Dr Paawan Wadhawan and Kajal Bhatia for their contributions to the project.

A big thanks to Kuntal Joisher, Siddharth Shukla and P. Venkatraman for sharing their insights about bone health.

Can't thank Dr Mahesh Shah, Dr Saravanan and Dr Tushar Mehta enough, for their invaluable words of experience.

Shruti Thatte who generously provided her equipment and support that helped kickstart this project.

Swapnil Raje, who took time out to help ideate the comic characters and lend the pages a dash of humour and lighter side that the project really needed.

Foreword

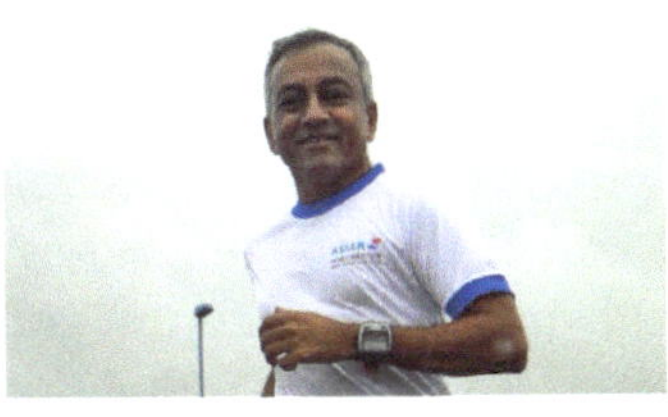

P Venkatraman, CA, Author & Marathon Runner

If I announced that I was going to abstain from bananas and green leafy vegetables, no one would be alarmed. And I would never be questioned about how I would get magnesium or be reminded that magnesium is essential for assimilating calcium into the bones. But if I said that I was abstaining from animal milk, eyebrows would go up and everybody would ask questions like, "How will you get your calcium?" or "What about your bone strength?". That is the power of the dairy industry lobbying over mass media, which the farmers unfortunately lack.

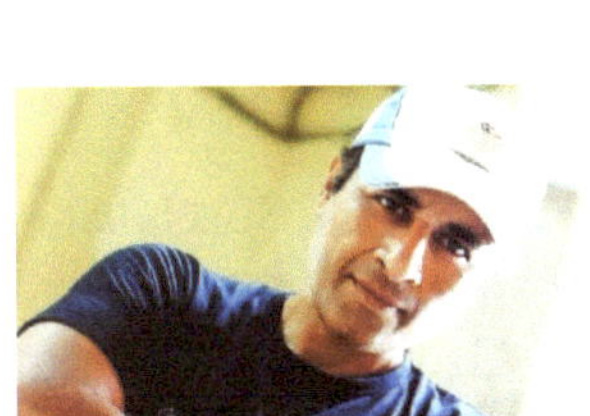

Siddharth Shukla, India's First Vegan Iron Man

Calcium can only be derived from animal-based dairy milk–is a big myth that has been busted by medical and scientific research. This book is an eye-opener for all as the writer herself is a well-known doctor. A must-read to clarify all your doubts concerning dairy consumption and bone health. Moreover, you will learn amazing recipes for improving overall wellbeing as well. Also, as long as we consume only plant-based foods, we get all the nutrients that we require–this is nature's arrangement. So we should not be misled by advertisements.

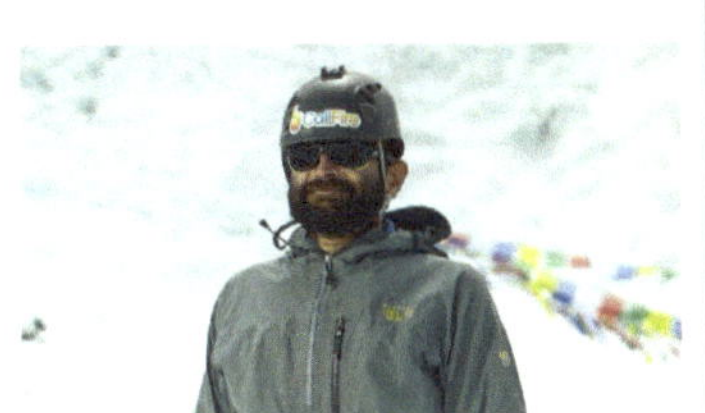

Kuntal Joisher, World's First Vegan Mountaineer Who Scaled Mt Everest twice

I was born and raised in a vegetarian family. However some 16 years ago, I turned vegan and sometime in 2010, I found my true calling–to climb Mt Everest–one of the toughest feats that would push one's body beyond its limits. I resolved to climb Everest as a vegan or not climb it at all. Finally, on 19 May 2016, I stood on the very top of Mt Everest after 45 days of hard climbing. My journey right up to that incredible day was extremely challenging and I realized that eating healthy vegan food supported my physical and mental fitness regime to a great extent. I was able to recover faster and push myself harder by doing increasingly more difficult workouts. My advice to everyone on a vegan lifestyle is to eat a healthy balanced diet, which is a good mix of fruits, vegetables, legumes, whole grains and finally, seeds and nuts. I get all my calcium from these foods, and don't use any supplements. Some of my favourite vegan calcium sources are–bananas, oranges, dates, sesame seeds, soymilk, tofu, beans and pulses.

Foreword

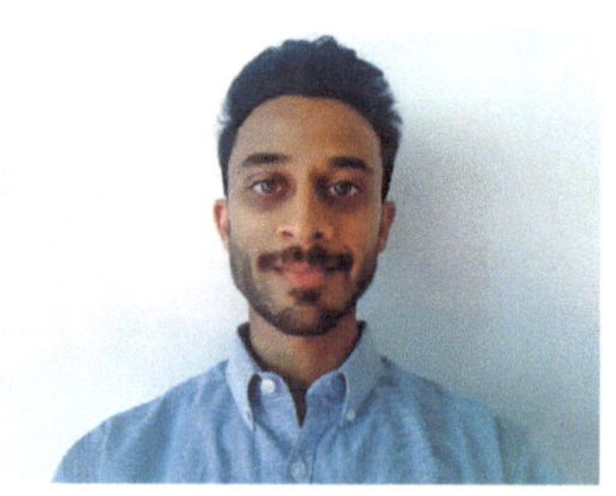

Dr Mahesh Shah MBBS, MRCGP, UK

"Cow's milk for strong bones!"-This the message fed to us from our earliest years. However, we have scientific data that animal products provide no bone protection and increase the risk of fractures, heart disease, diabetes and cancer, to name a few. Calcium indeed has an important role to play in bone health and other functions, and we can obtain this from natural whole plant foods, which also provide numerous other nutrients important for bone and general health. As we see from the healthiest populations in the world (called the Blue Zones), a plant-based diet along with exercise and other factors is integral to great health, happiness and longevity.

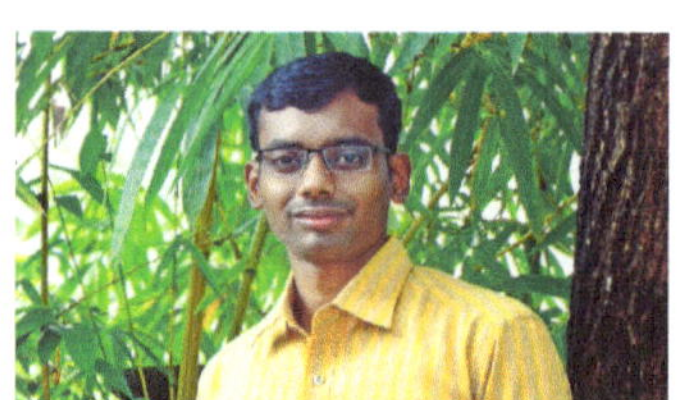

Dr Saravanan BHMS., PGDHSC., CLM., Nutrition& Lifestyle Medicine Specialist

Calcium is an important mineral needed for bone health. There are good plant-based sources of calcium that are far healthier than dairy products. Also, calcium present in plant-based foods can be easily absorbed by the body. We also need Vitamin D for calcium absorption and retention, which can be easily obtained from at least 15-20 minutes of daily sunlight exposure. Those who live in low temperature regions and have Vit D deficiency may need supplementation. Plant-based Vitamin D3 supplements are now available. A healthy plant-based diet can meet the calcium needs of every age group.

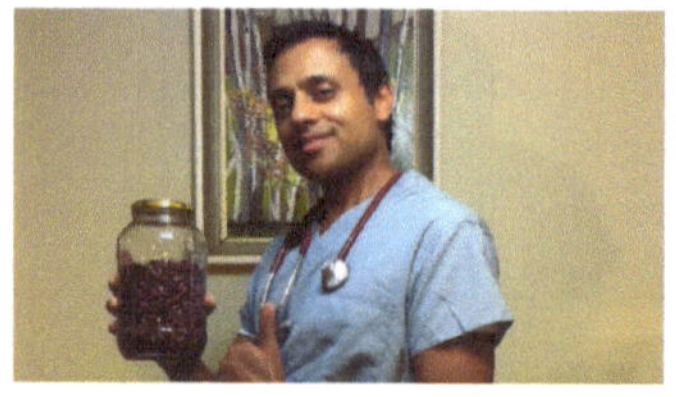

Dr Tushar Mehta MD, Family & Emergency Physician, Canada

Calcium intake is vital for bone health, so pay attention to the best sources outlined in this book. Also remember, the protein from pulses and especially soy combine with calcium to create healthy bones and prevent fractures. Get your exercise and eat fresh fruits and vegetables. The full combination is important!

Preface

The turning point of my life was in 2008, when I decided to give up dairy for 30 days and see what happens. Although I was a sceptic at first, I was astonished when my chronic migraine headaches & hyperacidity that I was suffering from for the past 18 years completely disappeared! This opened my eyes to a whole new world of holistic healing and I chose to give up dairy for life. I started researching all about dairy and discovered that whole & plant-based foods (wpbf) also help reverse lifestyle diseases. Since then, it has become my life's mission to create awareness about plant-based lifestyle for healthy living.

Over the years, I have held talks about whole and plant-based foods all over India and the world. I have also conducted many plant-based healthy cooking workshops and helped patients to reverse their diseases by following a plant-based lifestyle. Many of my articles on the healing power of wpbf have been published in prestigious newspapers and magazines as well. Encouraged by the palpable curiosity about "what", the next step was "how"–to smoothen the speedbumps of the transition. Thus in 2015, I penned "Dairy Alternatives" in English which was the 'need-of-the-moment' project for India. (Now this book is also published in Hindi and Gujarati.)

It has been 15 years since I gave up dairy products and I have never suffered from calcium deficiency or any other related condition. Same has been the experience of people all over the world. In fact, many have observed that their calcium levels actually improved once they gave up dairy products in their own lives. There are plant-based athletes, bodybuilders and sportsmen who are breaking all the adverse myths about plant-based nutrition. There are thousands across the globe who have reversed their lifestyle-related diseases like type 2 diabetes, hypertension, high cholesterol, obesity and heart diseases and are inspiring others to do the same. It is hard to go against the tide, but the strength comes from the very healthy foods that I have chosen to eat!

The journey continues.

'What About My Calcium?'

Every time I am asked this question, I can't help but smile. As soon as I advise my patients that the first step towards healthy living is to stop consuming dairy, I can always expect this question to pop up. Because of our cultural and religious associations with the use of dairy in our daily food habits, it is a challenge for many to give up dairy products. The common belief that comes down from earlier generations is that cow or buffalo milk is a "must for healthy bones, teeth and growth of an infant". Most people are skeptical about giving up dairy products for the fear of becoming fracture-prone if they give up dairy products.

Thus I decided to write this book to clear up the misconceptions about calcium and also create awareness that plants are super-sources of calcium. Also, it is about changing the mindset. It is the same source from where horses, bulls or elephants get their calcium. Earth is rich source of calcium and plants integrate that well. When we eat plants, we get our calcium as required.

Today, we are surrounded by a pandemic of lifestyle-related diseases and bone health is amongst the biggest health concerns to address right away. This is my humble effort to address some of these issues. The solution is to bring about a complete change in our food habits and to choose wpbf to not only reverse these diseases, but also to prevent them. You will need to take your own steps towards this lifestyle and this book will be very supportive on your journey. Wish you a very healthy life!

Disclaimer: This book is perhaps the first one-of-its-kind in the field of plant-based nutrition. However, I don't claim the book to be a nutrition guide, neither am I the final authority on this subject. I have provided a comprehensive chart of all the calcium-rich plant-based sources and presented nutrient-rich recipes that are rooted in our traditional Indian cuisine. However, I do not identify calcium as a separate mineral that we need. We live in the universe, connected with all minerals, which are required in variable quantities at different times and different stages in our lives. When we adopt a wpbf lifestyle, a big transformation happens. We start eating, relishing, absorbing, digesting and assimilating real foods which are a sum total of all macro- as well as micronutrients, followed by emotional fulfillment after each meal.

Dr Rupa Shah

How to use this book

Hello Readers! Welcome to my latest book 'What About My Calcium?'. You may be surprised to know that many common ingredients that we use for our daily cooking are actually rich sources of calcium. Try out a few recipes in this book and see how simple they are to make, and start integrating them in your daily meals. And although the book is aligned towards Indian cuisine, most of the ingredients are available globally and can be made by people all over the world.

In this book, we have included a comprehensive General Reference Guide to Calcium in Foods from **pg83** that enlists foods high on calcium across various categories i.e. from greens to grains. Additionally, we have over 40 delicious easy-to-make recipes starting from **pg25**. We have also explained symbols used to help you pick a recipe more suited for your requirements on **pg11**. The section also explains common terms often used in the book. This book is your handbook or kit to help empower your decisions right from the start point i.e. the produce market to your kitchen and finally the food on your plate.

Let's understand some terms and symbols that we have used in this book:

- **WFPD or WPBF:** We have altered the reference from whole foods & plant-based diet to **whole & plant -based foods**. Both include a broad spectrum of foods like vegetables, tubers, fruits, drinks, whole grains, cereals, and all foods sourced from plants. These foods are essentially eaten in whole food form. Wpbf excludes dairy, meat, fish and eggs.

- **Transition Foods (TF):** They are foods to enable beginners to faster transform their food choices by eliminating meat, fish, eggs and dairy products. Transition foods are NOT part of wpbf, but contain proteins and minerals as well. For instance, tea and coffee, cold-pressed oils, unrefined sugar, salt and other ingredients mentioned across this book. Once you have oriented yourself with the limitless and delicious options out there, then you can skip TF and shift to wpbf.

- **Jain Foods (JF):** These foods contain no garlic, ginger, potatoes, carrots or any roots. Many recipes labelled as 'JF' have mentioned garlic and ginger for taste, but they are optional and can be skipped.

How to use this book

Notes

1. **Preparation Time** mentioned in each recipe **Brief** box refers to the time taken to bring together all the individual ingredients for the respective recipe. It also includes **Soaking Time** of an ingredient before you start making the recipe or at times during the process as well.

2. Cook your food in vessels that are made of steel, iron and earthenware. Avoid cooking in aluminum or non-stick vessels.

3. Avoid using oil in your cooking. Use minimal amount of oil, or where required to grease the base of pans or plates.

How to use the Calcium Reference Table (Pg 83)

The book presents a General Calcium Reference Guide from Pg86 to enable you to make better choices from the produce and grocery market right down to transforming the food choices on your plate. Some of the values may not tally with nutritional values presented by other organizations, as there is no single gold standard of reference world over. We have made our best effort to present local whole foods which are often not found in international nutrition charts.

Just remember not to give too much importance to calcium values. Eat local, fresh, organic and seasonal foods often. Also consume local foods in rotation. There are counter-effects of eating too much of only one ingredient, so aim to eat a balanced meal. For instance, do not eat too many sesame seeds as it may lead to weight gain. Also, do not skip certain greens just because they have oxalates. These foods still contain other nutrients that your body needs. Finally, enjoy the food you eat, as this will help you assimilate it better and feel fulfilled after every meal.

The journey begins.

Legends

jf	Jain Food
gf	Gluten Free
nf	Nut Free
of	Oil Free
sof	Soy Free
suf	Sugar Free
wf	Whole Foods
nf	Transition Foods
tbsp	Tablespoon/Tablespoons
tsp	Teaspoons

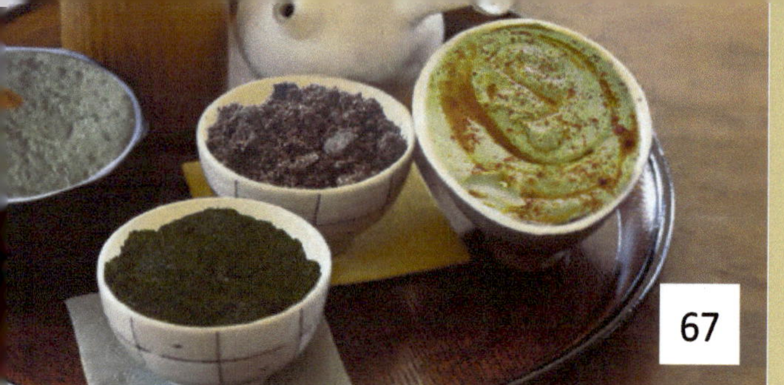

CONTENT

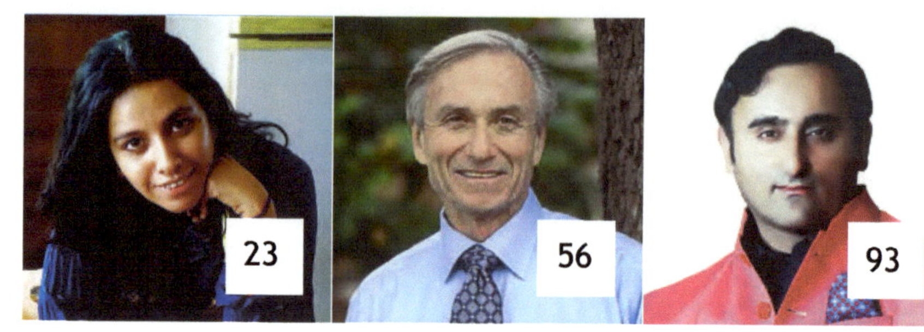

ENERAL REFERENCE GUIDE TO
CALCIUM IN FOODS
REEN LEAFY VEGETABLES
83

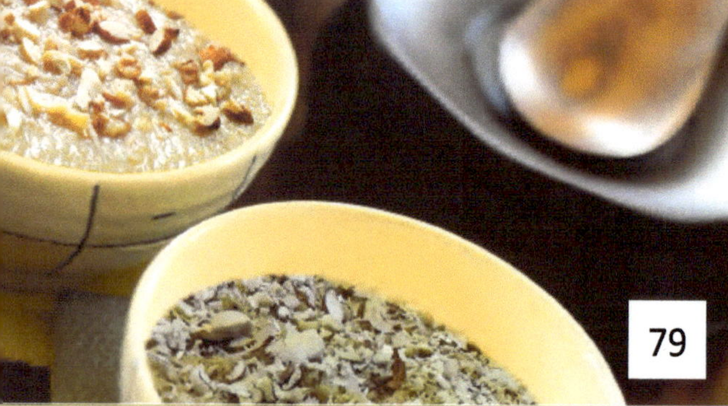

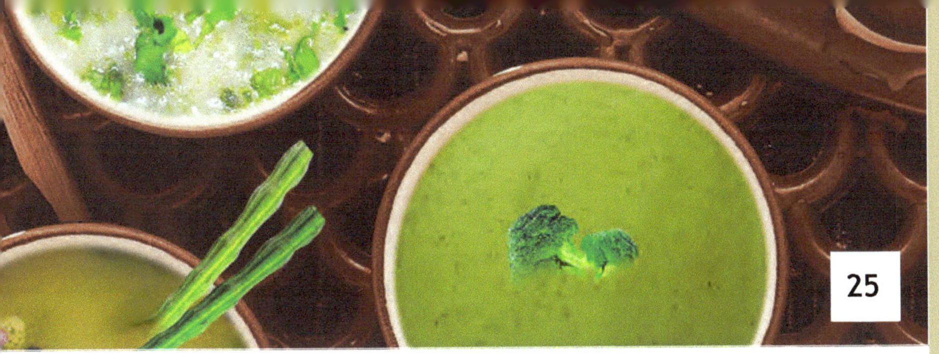

25

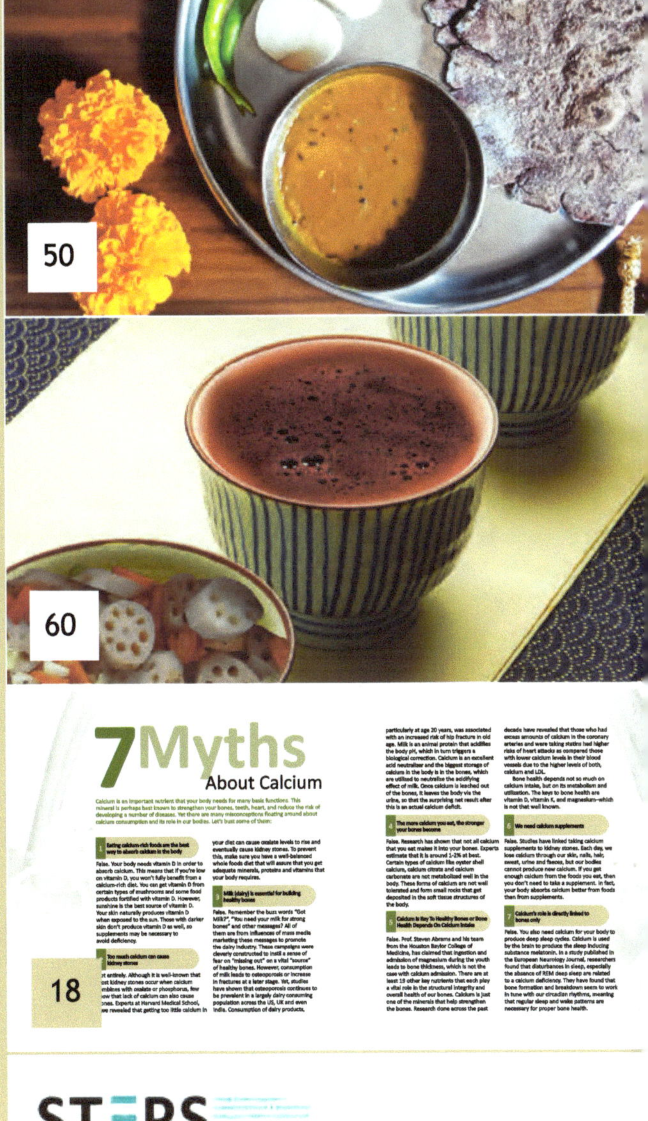

50
60
7Myths
About Calcium
18

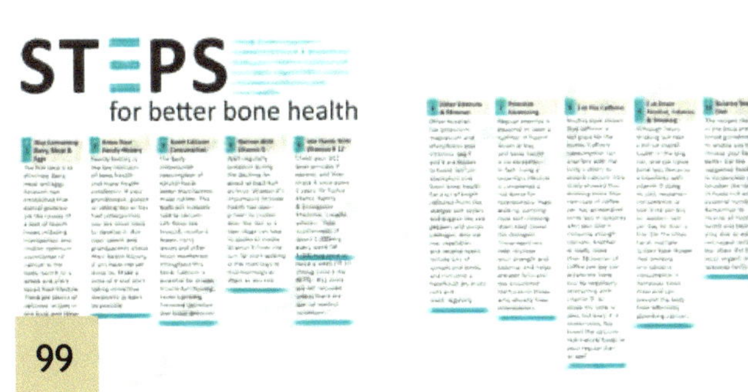

STEPS
for better bone health
99

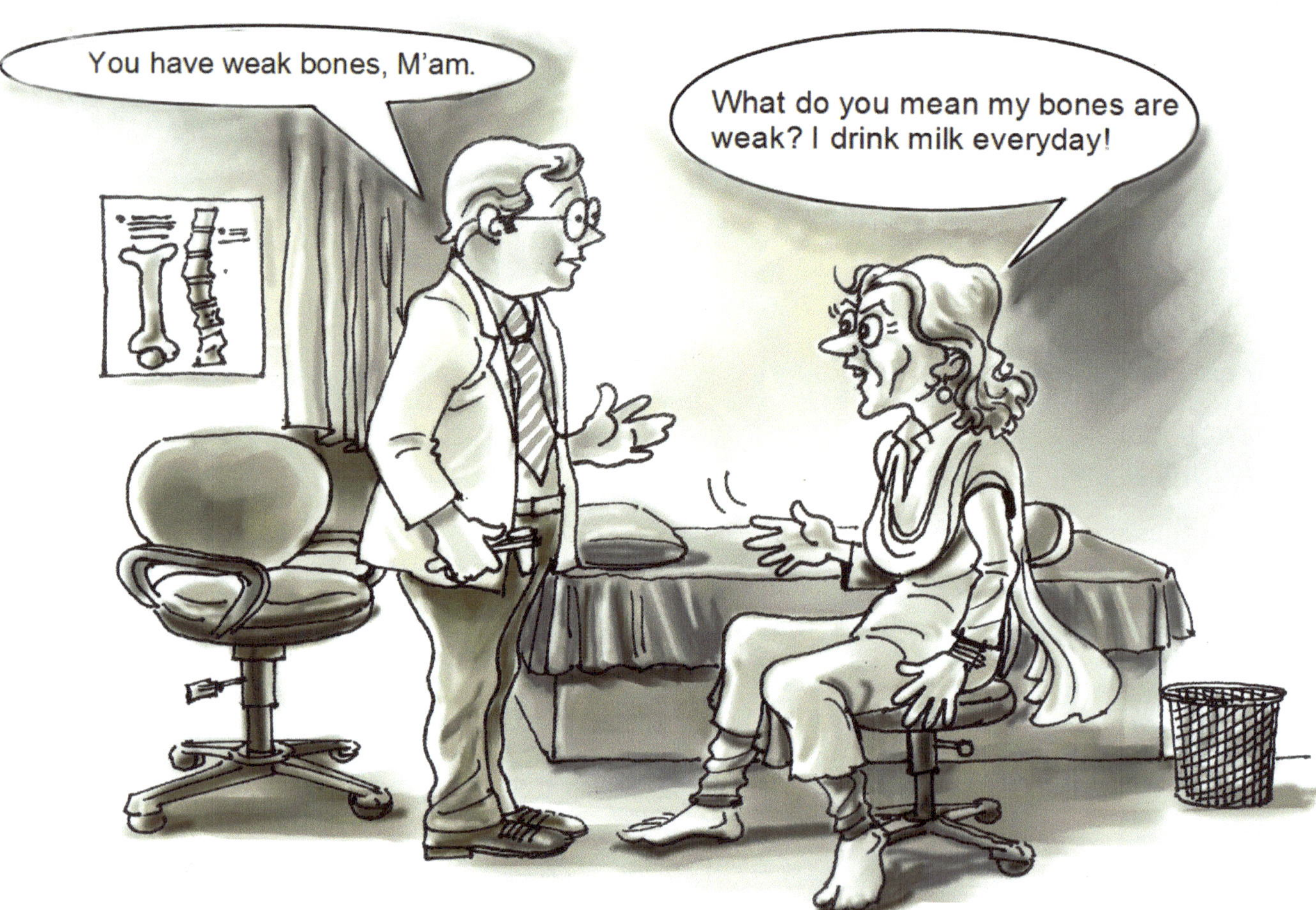
You have weak bones, M'am.
What do you mean my bones are weak? I drink milk everyday!

Quiz

How much do you know about calcium? Take this quiz and find out.

1. **What is the role of calcium in your body?**
   - ☐ Ensures muscles & nerves work properly
   - ☐ Builds healthy bones & teeth
   - ☐ Maintains blood pressure
   - ☐ All of the above

2. **You can get calcium from vegetables.**

   ☐ True ☐ False

3. **At what age does bone density naturally start to decline?**
   - ☐ From birth After age 30
   - ☐ After menopause Around age 60
   - ☐ Never

4. **The baby in the womb takes calcium from its mother.**

   ☐ True ☐ False

5. **Cutting down on calcium in your diet prevents kidney stones.**

   ☐ True ☐ False

6. **If you don't get enough calcium in your diet, your body will take the calcium it needs from your bones.**

   ☐ True ☐ False

7. **Who needs the most calcium?**
   - ☐ Children ages 4 to 8
   - ☐ Children and teens ages 10 to 20
   - ☐ Adults older than 50

8. **Your body needs one of the following to absorb calcium:**
   - ☐ Vitamin D Vitamin C Potassium

9. **You can consume supplements to prevent calcium deficiency.**

   ☐ True ☐ False

10. **The bigger the dose of calcium supplements, the more you absorb calcium.**

    ☐ True ☐ False

11. **It is possible to get too much calcium from un-natural sources.**

    ☐ True ☐ False

12. **Your bone mass and skeleton becomes weaker as you age.**

    ☐ True False

Answers

1. **What is the role of calcium in your body?**
   - Ensures muscles & nerves work properly
   - Builds healthy bones & teeth
   - Maintains blood pressure
   - **All of the above**

Ans: Most of you are aware that calcium plays the key role for strong bones and teeth. However, that is not all. Calcium is also required for muscles, nerves, and blood cells to function properly. Moreover, Harvard Health has reported that calcium is important for healthy blood pressure because it helps blood vessels tighten and relax when they need to.

2. **You can get calcium from vegetables.**
   - **True**

Ans: Greens like methi (fenugreek), Chinese cabbage, kale and broccoli are high on calcium. So are white and black sesame seeds. If you don't get enough calcium, you boost your chances of osteoporosis and arthritis.

3. **At what age does bone density naturally start to decline?**
   - **After age 30**

Ans: Bones start to weaken after hitting the age of 30, although you may not see the effects until later in life. It is never too early or too late to start bolstering your bone health with natural foods and regular outdoor exercises during the day.

4. **The baby in the womb takes calcium from its mother.**
   - **True**

Ans: The growing fetus or baby needs lots of calcium to grow its bones. It's especially important during the last 3 months. If you don't get enough calcium, the baby will get what it needs from your bones. Thus, when pregnant or breastfeeding, you need to eat calcium-rich foods. Also, any lost bone can be regained after giving birth or after breast-feeding.

5. **Cutting down on calcium in your diet prevents kidney stones.**
   - **False**

Ans: Most kidney stones are made of a type of calcium called calcium oxalate. The calcium in foods doesn't cause them. (But too much calcium from supplements may make kidney stones more likely.) Bottom line: Get the recommended amount of calcium—not too much, and not too little.

6. **If you don't get enough calcium in your diet, your body will take the calcium it needs from your bones.**
   - **True**

Ans: Your body procures calcium from the foods you eat. If you're not getting enough calcium, your body will leach the mineral from your bones.

7. **Who needs the most calcium?**
   - **Children and teens from ages 10 to 20**

Ans: Children and teens from ages 10 to 20 are growing quickly, and so are their bones. So they need a lot of calcium by including green leaves and sesame seeds in the foods every day.

8. **Your body needs one of the following to absorb calcium:**
   - **Vitamin D**

Ans: The body requires vitamin D to absorb calcium. Not getting enough vitamin D can increase your risk of osteoporosis. Remember, you cannot consume calcium alone. Ensure you are eating balanced whole foods and walking outdoors regularly, to expose yourself to the sunlight. Refer to **pg101** for more details about Vitamin D.

9. **You can consume supplements to prevent calcium deficiency.**
   - **False**

Ans: Avoid consuming calcium supplements. Your body can source all the calcium it requires from whole and plant-based foods.

10. **The bigger the dose of calcium supplements, the more you absorb calcium.**
    - **False**

Ans: You are now entering dangerous grounds. Do NOT take calcium supplements without consulting your doctor. Excessive dosage can lead to organ complications and disable your body from absorbing the required amounts. Excess calcium consumption will then be flushed out in your urine or can get deposited in your arteries, joints or kidneys causing kidney stone or thicken your arteries.

11. **It is possible to get too much calcium.**
    - **True**

Ans: High levels of calcium can cause calcification of the arteries, kidney issues and reduction in the absorption of minerals like iron and zinc. Do not self-subscribe calcium supplements. Remember, you can get all the calcium you need with a balanced whole and plant-based foods.

12. **Your bone mass and skeleton becomes weaker as you age.**
    - **True**

Ans: Yes, your bones become weaker as you age. To cut back on the loss of bone mass, ensure that you get enough calcium in your diet. You should also do weight-bearing exercise.

9-12 Answers Are Correct

Great! Congratulations! You are well informed and have your facts right! You can skip directly to the **Recipe Section** from **pg 27** and get kitchen savvy, or read on to test your knowledge about whether you are aware about the lesser known details about calcium in the following pages. Keep it up!

5-8 Correct

Well Done! You are well on your way to learning all you need to know about calcium in your practical life. Flip through the following chapter that busts many myths about calcium and enables you to stay on top of your health.

Below 5 Correct

Get Going! If you are new to the world of whole and plant-based foods, you could not have picked a better time to begin your journey. NOW is the time. You can re-do the test to bone-up your knowledge about calcium, or take a break and try it later.

7Myths
About Calcium

Calcium is an important nutrient that your body needs for many basic functions. This mineral is perhaps best known to strengthen your bones, teeth, heart, and reduce the risk of developing a number of diseases. Yet there are many misconceptions floating around about calcium consumption and its role in our bodies. Let's bust some of them:

1 Eating calcium-rich foods are the best way to absorb calcium in the body

False. Your body needs vitamin D in order to absorb calcium. This means that if you're low on vitamin D, you won't fully benefit from a calcium-rich diet. You can get vitamin D from certain types of mushrooms and some food products fortified with vitamin D. However, sunshine is the best source of vitamin D. Your skin naturally produces vitamin D when exposed to the sun. Those with darker skin don't produce vitamin D as well, so supplements may be necessary to avoid deficiency.

2 Too much calcium can cause kidney stones

Not entirely. Although it is well-known that most kidney stones occur when calcium combines with oxalate or phosphorus, few know that lack of calcium can also cause stones. Experts at Harvard Medical School have revealed that getting too little calcium in your diet can cause oxalate levels to rise and eventually cause kidney stones. To prevent this, make sure you have a well-balanced whole foods diet that will assure that you get adequate minerals, proteins and vitamins that your body requires.

3 Milk (dairy) is essential for building healthy bones

False. Remember the buzz words "Got Milk?", "You need your milk for strong bones" and other messages? All of them are from influences of mass media marketing these messages to promote the dairy industry. These campaigns were cleverly constructed to instill a sense of fear on "missing out" on a vital "source" of healthy bones. However, consumption of milk leads to osteoporosis or increase in fractures at a later stage. Yet, studies have shown that osteoporosis continues to be prevalent in a largely dairy consuming population across the US, UK and even India. Consumption of dairy products, particularly at age 20 years, was associated with an increased risk of hip fracture in old age. Milk is an animal protein that acidifies the body pH, which in turn triggers a biological correction. Calcium is an excellent acid neutralizer and the biggest storage of calcium in the body is in the bones, which are utilized to neutralize the acidifying effect of milk. Once calcium is leached out of the bones, it leaves the body via the urine, so that the surprising net result after this is an actual calcium deficit.

4 The more calcium you eat, the stronger your bones become

False. Research has shown that not all calcium that you eat makes it into your bones. Experts estimate that it is around 1-2% at best. Certain types of calcium like oyster shell calcium, calcium citrate and calcium carbonate are not metabolized well in the body. These forms of calcium are not well tolerated and form small rocks that get deposited in the soft tissue structures of the body.

5 Calcium is Key to Healthy Bones or Bone Health Depends on Calcium Intake

False. Prof. Steven Abrams and his team from the Houston Baylor College of Medicine, has claimed that ingestion and admission of magnesium during the youth leads to bone thickness, which is not the case with calcium admission. There are at least 19 other key nutrients that each play a vital role in the structural integrity and overall health of our bones. Calcium is just one of the minerals that help strengthen the bones. Research done across the past decade have revealed that those who had excess amounts of calcium in the coronary arteries and were taking statins had higher risks of heart attacks as compared those with lower calcium levels in their blood vessels due to the higher levels of both, calcium and LDL.

Bone health depends not so much on calcium intake, but on its metabolism and utilization. The keys to bone health are vitamin D, vitamin K, and magnesium–which is not that well known.

6 We need calcium supplements

False. Studies have linked taking calcium supplements to kidney stones. Each day, we lose calcium through our skin, nails, hair, sweat, urine, and feces, but our bodies cannot produce new calcium. If you get enough calcium from the foods you eat, then you don't need to take a supplement. In fact, your body absorbs calcium better from foods than from supplements.

7 Calcium's role is directly linked to bones only

False. You also need calcium for your body to produce deep sleep cycles. Calcium is used by the brain to produce the sleep inducing substance melatonin. In a study published in the European Neurology Journal, researchers found that disturbances in sleep, especially the absence of REM deep sleep are related to a calcium deficiency. They have found that bone formation and breakdown seem to work in tune with our circadian rhythms, meaning that regular sleep and wake patterns are necessary for proper bone health.

About Calcium

Calcium is one of the key elements and required for all life on earth. It represents the living structure of our bodies, not just the bones and teeth. Calcium may also be said to represent voltage in an electrical analogy. In fact, the mineral regulates the voltage at which nerve cells fire.

Too much bio unavailable calcium and too little available calcium will prevent the proper firing of the nerve cells. The imbalance can cause mental and physical depression, among other symptoms. It also impairs the passage of nutrients and waste or creates thyroid complications. It is important to note that the balance of calcium, and its bioavailability, is really the key to health in all living things. Calcium is also used to neutralize high acidity in the blood.

Dr L Wilson, MD, US, states that calcium exerts a kind of pressure that allows life to flourish on earth. Without it, life cannot exist. As one's calcium stores are used up, life ebbs out of the body. As one replaces the body's calcium properly, life energy returns. In this regard, calcium functions as a kind of valve or receiver of etheric energy that fuels the human, animal and even the plant frame or organism.

Criti-Cal Tips

Calcium is often misunderstood for its role in our bodies. Minerals like Magnesium, Chlorine & Hydrochloric Acid, Potassium, Copper and Vitamin A are some of the minerals that we need to consume to better synergize or boost the absorption of calcium in our bodies.

Just as there are elements in food consumption that can enable us to effectively absorb calcium in our bodies, there are other ingredients that can upset its balance in our bodies, such as any form of dairy, refined sugar, sweet chocolates, caffeine, coffee, lead, fluoride, which are mostly founds in high-processed foods. Also over-dependency on drugs like antibiotics, corticosteroids, steroids, tetracycline, antacids and aspirin are only some of the meds that inhibit calcium absorption in our bodies.

Some calcium-rich foods also contain oxalates (green leaves) and phytates (seeds, bean, legumes & grains), both of which can bind together with calcium and other minerals to inhibit the amount of calcium that we absorb. However, there is a way out. Boil a high-oxalate food like spinach to reduce its oxalate content. Moreover, the best way to reduce the phytate content in foods is to sprout them.

It is important to note that lack of regular exercise and not enough stress management also leads to increased calcium loss. Finally, for women, blood loss and hormonal tips during menses cause natural calcium loss. Which is why it's important to build blood after the cycle.

Studies on calcium supplements in the recent years have suggested that if consumed in excess, it can lead to health complications. In the study, 'Risk of High Dietary Calcium for Arterial Calcification in Older Adults' by John JB Anderson and Philip J Klemmer, they found that when calcium intake consistently exceeds the RDA (Recommended Dietary Allowances) of older adults, or when a substantial amount of the calcium is derived from calcium supplements, it "may accelerate arterial calcification and raise the risk of cardiovascular events." The study advises that health professionals need to continue monitoring calcium recommendations, especially when calcium is consumed from non-food sources.

Calcium Supplementation Is Not Natural

A study has found that calcium supplements did not reduce hip fracture risk among people who consumed calcium supplements, but rather an increased risk was possible. Given these findings, individuals should be discouraged from taking calcium supplements and advised to obtain calcium from their diet instead. Scientists have found that "our body is not stupid"–If we eat less calcium, our body absorbs more and excretes less, and if we eat more calcium, we absorb less and excrete more to stay in balance. This is also confirmed by Dr T Colin Campbell in his book 'Whole…'[10], where he states, "The percentage of calcium absorbed can vary by at least two-fold; the higher the calcium intake, the lower the proportion absorbed into the blood, ensuring adequate calcium for the body and no more." This may explain why in most studies, no relationship has been found between calcium intake from food and bone loss anywhere in the skeleton because the body just seems to take care of it.

Supplements Don't Reduce Fracture Risk

A review published in the Annals of Internal Medicine has found that there's no evidence to support the idea that calcium and vitamin D supplements prevent falls and bone fractures in older adults. After two systematic evidence reviews and a meta-analysis on the health effects of vitamin D supplements, researchers from the United States Preventive Services Task Force found no evidence that daily supplementation prevented bone fractures, though it did increase a patient's risk of kidney stones. Dr Rupa Shah states, "We do not recommend calcium supplements to our patients. Instead, we encourage all to source their calcium from a balanced whole food lifestyle."

Excess Calcium Effects

Bones are made of at least 12 different minerals, not just calcium – and excess calcium and a lack of other essential minerals can actually lead to an increased risk of fractures. Excess calcium in our bodies has huge metabolic effects leading to a host of medical problems.

In the study, 'The Nurses' Health Study' of 122,000 women, which analyzed the risk factors for major chronic diseases, women with the highest calcium consumption from dairy products actually had substantially more fractures than women who drank less milk.

Prevention of osteoporosis is the best course of action. The more physically active you are early in life, the lower your risk of osteoporosis. And the more exercises you do, at any stage in life i.e. walking, running, yoga and any activity that keeps you on your feet, the lower the risk.

In fact, there is so much calcium in the foods we commonly eat (like green leaves, sesame seeds, and added calcium in everything from juices to cereals and protein bars), most of us are already overloaded even before we think of taking a supplement. In the best of all worlds, dietary calcium and the calcium supplements our doctors insist we take, cause a mineral imbalance that can have disastrous results.

Down To The Bone

The bones in our bodies consist of a living network of protein fibres, which keeps our bones elastic and flexible. These fibres create the framework upon which mineral crystals of calcium phosphate salts are set. The living protein fibres help make the bone flexible while the mineral calcium salts, which are dead, make the bone hard, dense and heavy.

Bones are constantly dissolving and rebuilding by specialized cells within us. All our bones renew themselves every seven to ten years completely. Bone loss that can lead to osteoporosis happens when the activity of the bone-dissolving cells predominates over that of the bone-building cells.

Calcium's role goes beyond just building bones and cartilages. It is also useful for relaxing muscles and preventing muscle spasm. Dr Gabriel Cousens, MD, USA, says, "Calcium is important for the flow of electrical energy in the system, and it combines with phosphate intracellularly and extracellularly to form an alkaline compound, calcium phosphate. Ionic calcium is an extremely important transport mineral for bringing other nutrients into the cell."

The Aging Process

After mid-life, the loss of the elasticity of the protein fibre bone network increases the risk of fractures. These losses are caused by the gradual withdrawal of our etheric life forces from our bones with aging. However, it is only when the life forces withdraw at a faster than average rate for our age that osteoporosis and an abnormally high risk of fractures come about. Yet, the integrity and flexibility of this living framework are the most important factors protecting us from fractures.

To avoid fractures and to have healthy and strong, quick-healing bones we must learn how to maintain the tightness and the resilience of the living protein fibres that are deposited within that protein fibre framework. Osteoporosis is not just the loss of bone mineral mass (calcium crystals), but also the fraying of the intimate fabric of living protein fibres which forms the very basis of our bones. Modern research has confirmed that vegetables, leafy greens, and whole grains like oats, rye and brown rice, are rich in the nutrients needed by our inner building cells, which are our etheric life forces, to build a strong protein fibre bone matrix and to calcify it into sturdy and flexible bones.

Many of the causes of osteoporosis mentioned across this book help create an acidic inner environment. It can also be triggered by stress, nervousness, exhaustion, excessive exercise and by an overactive thyroid gland. All of these factors increase the tendency to osteoporosis by depleting our vital etheric forces. When our life forces are strong and our stress is low, our inner environment becomes alkaline and we slow down and relax. Many of our modern illnesses, including osteoporosis, stem from dietary and lifestyle influences that speed us up, make us inwardly acidic and brittle and deplete our etheric vitality.

The Real Backbone

Dr Cousens in his website, 'treeoflifecenterus.com' explains: Calcium is responsible for solidity, as well as movement. Without sufficient calcium in the body, we end up with defective teeth and poor bone metabolism. It is important for digestion, is a great alkalinizer, and promotes growth and vitality. It also helps with the clotting mechanism to prevent haemorrhaging. Calcium acts to calm the nerves, neutralize stomach acidity, and protect against nervous exhaustion. It helps to strengthen the walls of the arteries and veins. The muscles require appropriate calcium to work correctly.'

The importance of calcium cannot be emphasized enough. But for calcium to be optimally utilized, we need foods that are high in sodium and chlorine. "When there is an imbalance of calcium in relationship to sodium, there is a tendency for a general hardening of the body, which is known as calcification. So an excess of calcium, or a deficiency of sodium, can create a precipitation of calcium in the tissues", points out Dr Cousens.

Calcium plays a role in building personality traits as well. Calcium deficiency can also affect the power of memory and influence personality traits. For instance, a calcium deficiency can create qualities of selfishness, subtle antisocial qualities in the personality. It may also cause depression, melancholy, mental confusion, and dull feeling in the head, as well as softening of bones, weak teeth, and tooth decay. Calcium deficiencies show up with symptoms of weakness, fear, indecision, lack of will power, tendency to haemorrhage, cramps in the calves, vein fatigue, digestive problems, soft bones, rickets, scurvy and tuberculosis. The deficiency of calcium has a long list of issues, but that is the case with any kind of imbalance in our body. Our bodies can get the required minerals from a balanced diet of whole and plant-based foods. Once we work towards a healthy lifestyle that includes regular exercise, we do not have to worry about any type of deficiency.

References

1. *Harvard Women's Health Watch*
2. *http://treeoflifecenterus.com/calcium/ (Dr Gabriel Cousens' Blog)*
3. *www.nutritionfacts.org by Dr Michael Greger*
4. *http://www.naturalhealthprotocol.com/calcium.html*
5. *https://www.ncbi.nlm.nih.gov/pmc/articles/PMC3820054/*
6. *https://www.everydayhealth.com/womens-health-photos/health-risks-of-calcium-supplements.aspx#02*
7. *http://www.anthromed.org/Article.aspx?artpk=351*
8. *https://drlwilson.com/Articles/calcium.htm*
9. *http://aprilcrowell.com/asian-medicine/calcium-one-cool-mineral/*
10. *'Whole: Rethinking The Science of Nutrition' by Dr T Colin Campbell*

> “It takes more than just calcium to build, maintain and repair bones.”

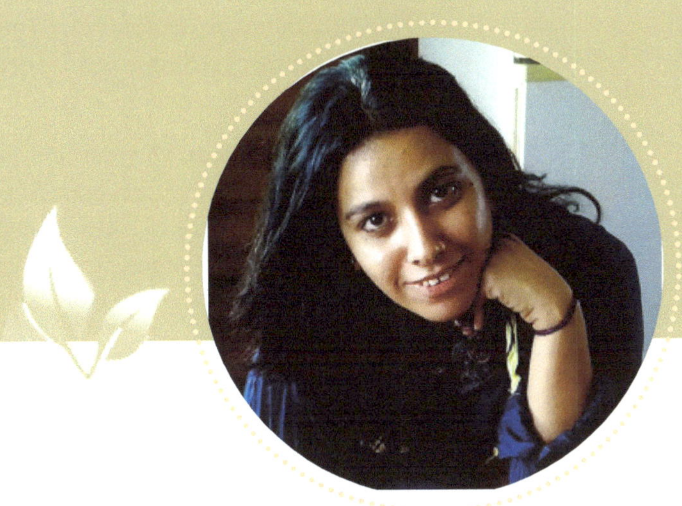

Kajal Bhatia On Calcium

Whole Food Nutrition, BSc (FSN) & CDE

Kajal is a Whole-Food Nutritionist and a Diabetes educator. An exponent of natural health and wellness, she is also a health food forager. She pursued Nutrition as a major at BMN College and SNDT University, Mumbai. And followed up with a diabetes educator expertise. She is currently pursuing a Doctorate program in United States for whole food sciences

What can be the one statement to help us clear the fog about calcium consumption?

Calcium does not come from milk alone; there are better absorbable plant sources of calcium.

Is calcium related to weight gain or weight loss?

Calcium does not have any significant measurable effect on weight loss nor is it associated with weight gain.

Is ‘Calcium Deficiency’ in an urban diet a myth or a reality?

Calcium deficiency is increasingly becoming a reality, despite awareness about calcium and its importance for bone health. This is due to the lack of information around calcium. Importance of other micro-minerals along with Vitamin D in the formation of bones is often misunderstood or ignored. Despite having a number of calcium supplements, osteoporosis causes more than 8.9 million fractures annually according to a result study published in International Osteoporosis Foundation.

(Ref: https://www.iofbonehealth.org/facts-statistics#category-14)

According to you, what aspect of calcium consumption is most misunderstood?

Just calcium builds bones. Ignorance or lack of awareness about how bones require phosphorous, magnesium, potassium along with Vit D is a largely ignored fact.

Do women require more calcium dosage as compared to men, especially post-menopause?

Calcium requirements for women go up post-menopause due to estrogen deficit as a result of no menstrual cycle. The requirements also increase during pregnancy and lactation.

Please elaborate on the minerals required by the body to sustain bone health.

It takes more than just calcium to build, maintain and repair bones. Phosphorous, zinc, magnesium & potassium are also the essential micro-minerals needed to support bone formation, resorption and their maintenance. These too are components of the bone structure. Vitamin D also helps as an ally assisting the body to absorb calcium from foods.

At what age should one take the first Bone Density test and Serum Calcium test?

Bone Density Test: One can consider testing bone density in any of the following cases:

- You are a woman age 65 or older
- You are a man age 70 or older
- You break a bone after age 50
- You are a woman with a menopausal age with risk factors
- You are a post-menopausal woman
- Under age 65 with risk factors
- You are a man age 50-69 with risk factors.
- Constant back-pain, joint pain, lack of energy

(Ref: National Osteoporosis Foundation- https:// www.nof.org/patients/diagnosis-information/bone-density-examtesting/)

Serum Calcium Test: One can get Serum Calcium tested at any age irrespective of presence of any bone issue/ disorder, as it is a very commonly performed clinical test to determine calcium levels in the blood.

And at what frequency or intervals should one take re-tests after the first base-line test?

Bone Density tests can be repeated every two years while Serum Calcium can be tested twice a year or annually.

Can you advise how to strengthen bones and teeth? Also suggest a meal plan for those who are just starting on whole & plant-based foods.

Tips to strengthen bones and teeth:

- Avoid acidic foods.
- Reduce junk intake for more minerals to be absorbed and utilized.
- Increase intake of natural plant-based calcium sources such as almonds, sesame, oranges, spinach, potato, amaranth, figs, ragi, dry coconut, colocassia leaves (patra) and palm jaggery.
- Spend more time in the morning sun.
- Chew more.

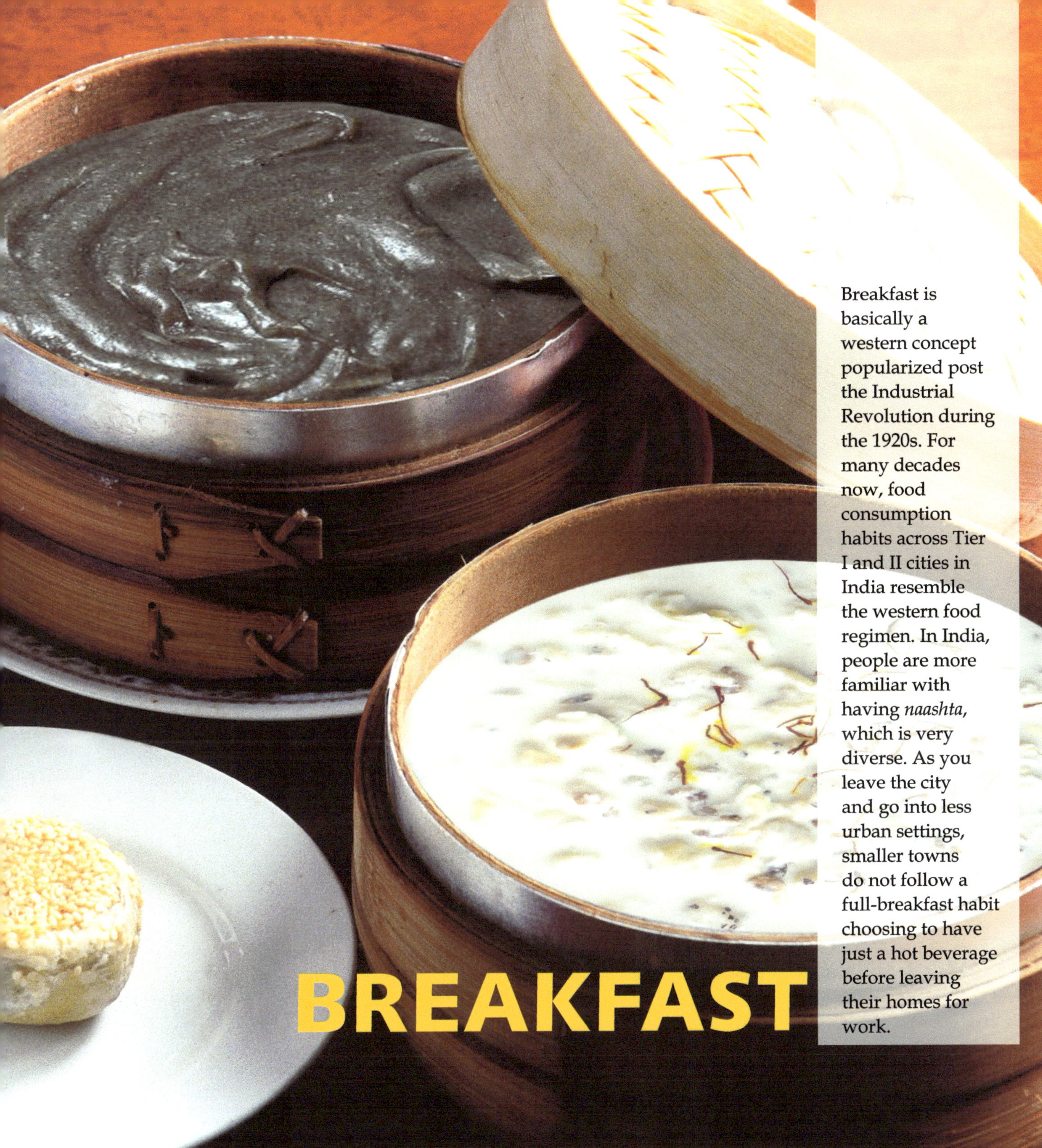

BREAKFAST

Breakfast is basically a western concept popularized post the Industrial Revolution during the 1920s. For many decades now, food consumption habits across Tier I and II cities in India resemble the western food regimen. In India, people are more familiar with having *naashta,* which is very diverse. As you leave the city and go into less urban settings, smaller towns do not follow a full-breakfast habit choosing to have just a hot beverage before leaving their homes for work.

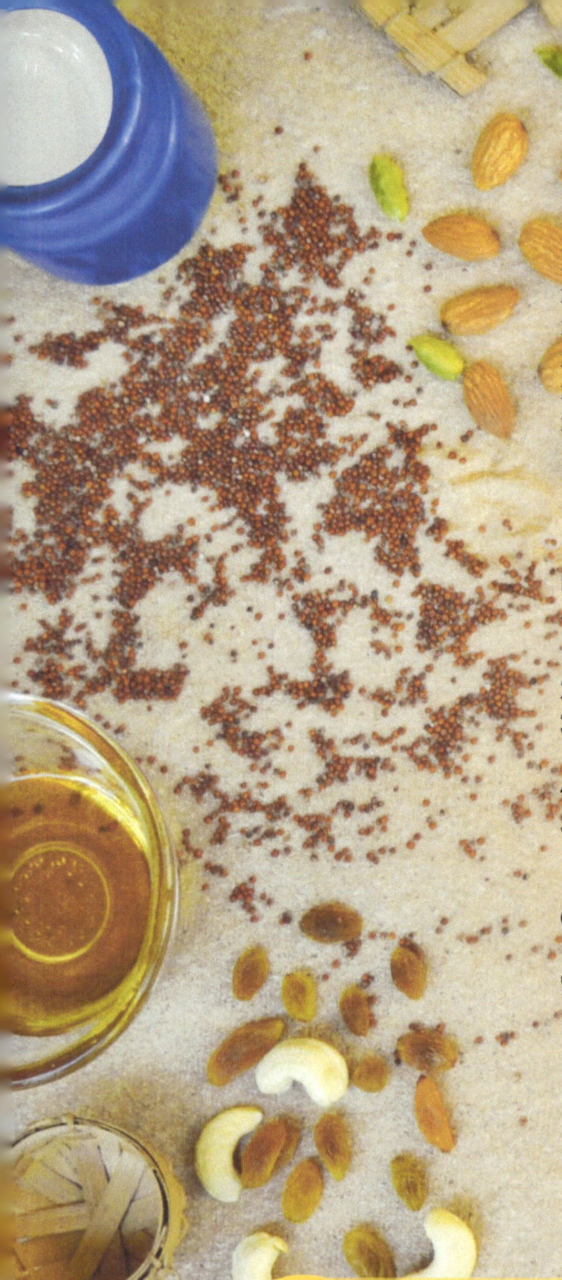

NACHANI (RAGI) OR FINGER-MILLET PORRIDGE

Nachani or Ragi *(Finger-Millets)* is a powerhouse of health-benefiting nutrients that help in reducing weight. The grain is a very rich source of minerals. It has been found to have between 5-30 times the calcium content found in other cereals. The grain is also rich in phosphorus, potassium and iron. It is easy to cook even as a healthy mono meal and makes excellent meals for children and pregnant women.

jf gf sof of 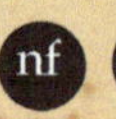 nf 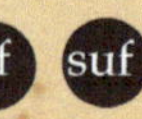 suf wf

Ingredients

1. Split Nachani *(Finger-Millets)* Grains (1/4 Cup)
2. Water (1 1/4 Cup)
3. Non-Dairy Milk* (Soy or Almond Milk etc. / 1/2 Cup)
4. Cardamom Powder (1/4 Tsp)
5. Natural Sweetener* (Date Syrup/ Raisin Paste/ Jaggery Powder / Raw Sugar/ 2 Tbsp)
6. Rock Salt or Unprocessed Sea Salt (1 Pinch)
7. Chopped Nuts & Dry Fruits for garnishing Like Almonds, Pistachio, Cashews, Walnuts & Raisins (Few of Each)

BRIEF

Preparation (Soaking)
Time: **8-10 Hours**
No. Of Servings: **1 Cup**
Fridge Life: **1 Day**

Method

- Wash nachani grains well with water.
- Take a bowl and add nachani as well as 1/4 cup fresh water. Leave it covered for minimum of 8 hours and maximum of 10 hours. This will soften up the nachani grains. Drain the water.
- Blend the grains well with 1 cup water in a blender. Using a stone grinder is the best way. The nachani milk is ready. No need to strain. This way, you can extract about 1 cup nachani milk.
- Take a broad pan and start cooking the milk on low flame for 10 minutes, constantly stirring the milk to make sure that there are no lumps formed and the milk mixture is evenly cooked.
- After cooking for 5 minutes, add ½ cup non-dairy milk. Continue cooking the mixture on low flame while stirring.
- Add 2 Tbsp of a natural sweetener
- Add a pinch of salt and cardamom powder.
- In 10 minutes, the mixture will turn thick.
- Garnish with chopped nuts/dry fruits.

RAJGIRA (AMARANTH) PUFFS PORRIDGE IN ALMOND MILK

A yummy morning treat and can be a great motivation for the kids to get out of bed. Rajgira puffs are nutrient-rich for growing children as well as senior citizens. They make a wholesome ready-to-eat breakfast option.

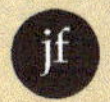
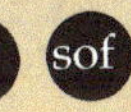
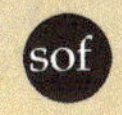
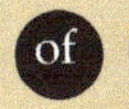
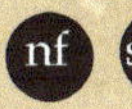
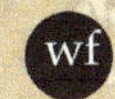

jf gf sof of nf suf wf

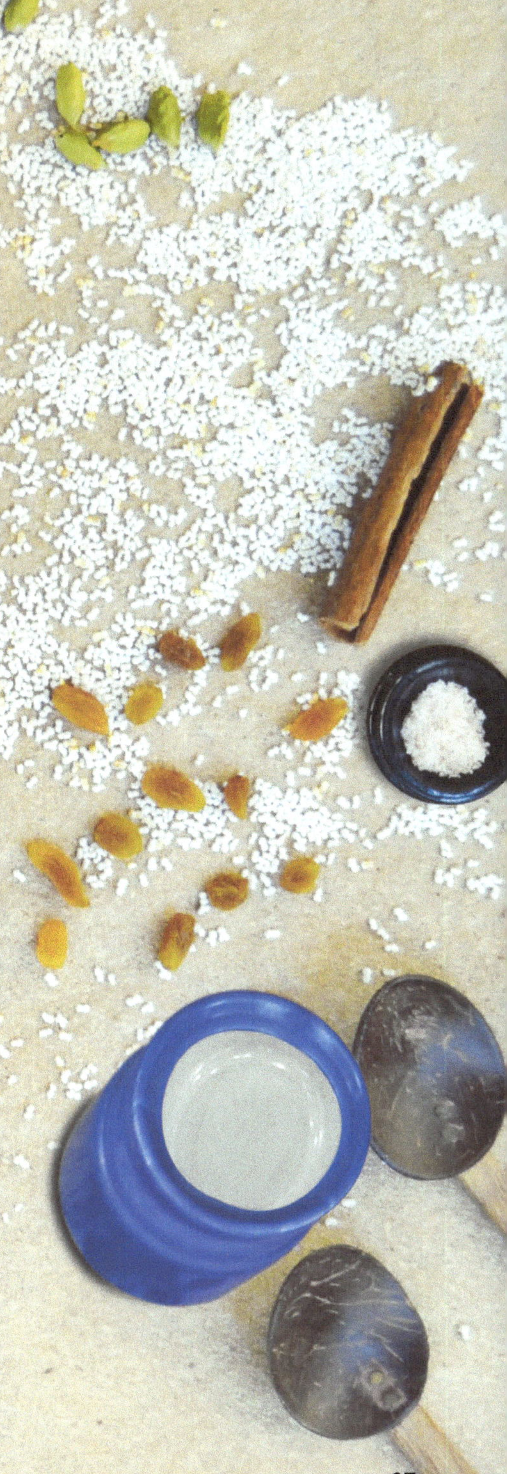

Ingredients

1. Rajgira *(Amaranth)* Puffs (6 Tbsp)
2. Almond Milk* (¾ Cup)
3. Raisins (10 Pc/ Semi-Crushed)
4. Rock Salt (Pinch)
5. Crushed Cardamom (Pinch)

Method

- Add rajgira puffs in the almond milk.
- Add raisins, cardamom and salt as well. Stir well. The puffs will soak up most of the almond milk, while the raisins will add sweetness.
- Ready to serve.

Tip: Alternatively, you can add cinnamon.

Tip: Raisins are healthier than white sugar, while a pinch of salt enhances the taste of the porridge.

* *For dairy-free milk recipes, refer to '**Dairy Alternatives**' by Dr Rupa Shah, available on amazon.in and healthrevolution.in.*

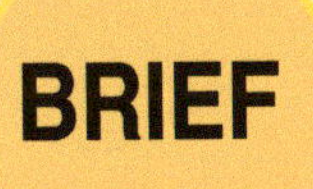

BRIEF

Preparation (Soaking) Time: **5 Min**
Preparation Time: **2 Min**
Cooking Time: **Not Required**
No. Of Servings: **1 Cup**
Fridge Life: **1 Day**

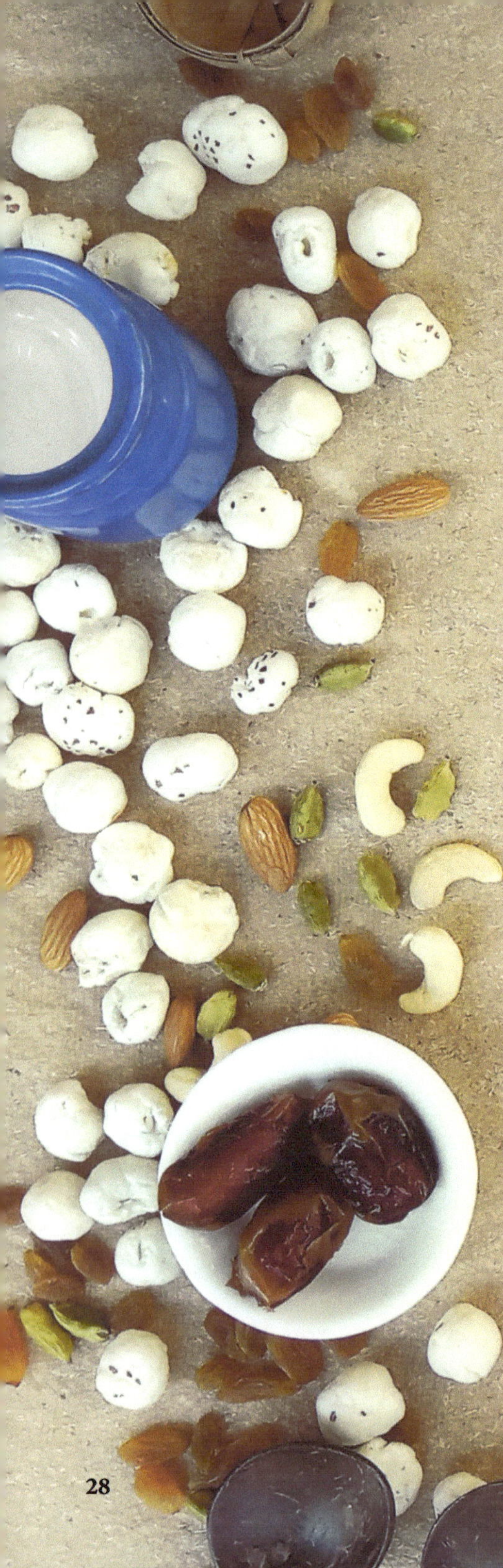

MAKHANA (WATER LILY) KHEER

Makhana is a healthier breakfast option, compared to cereals and popcorn. Unfortunately this crop is slowly being phased out by farmers who cultivate these in the central wetlands. Farmers have reduced growing makhana due to reduced demand from consumers. The reduced demand can be attributed to the heavy influence of big corporate advertising of food giants that have changed our food habits. Makhanas are delicious and although this recipe is usually made during fasting periods, it can also make a flavourful dessert.

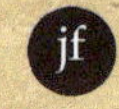

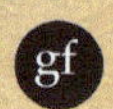

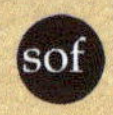

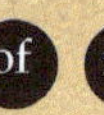

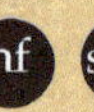

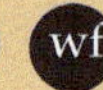

wf

Ingredients

1. Makhana (*Water Lily Seeds*) (1 Cup)
2. Dairy-Free Milk (1/2 Litre)
3. Mixed Nuts (2 Tbsp/Chopped Almonds & Pistachios)
4. Dates or Raisins Syrup (4 Tbsps. or As Per Taste)
5. Cardamom Powder (1 Tsp)

Method

- Cut the makhanas into small halves.
- Roast them for 5 minutes.
- Boil soy or almond milk in a vessel for 5 minutes.
- When the milk starts boiling, add the makhana
- On a low flame, keep cooking on stove for about 15 minutes.
- Add nuts and cardamom powder.
- Add any natural sweetener if desired. It will become thick in consistency.
- It can be served hot or chilled.

Tip: Stir often so that it does not stick to the bottom of the pan

BRIEF

Preparation Time: **10 Min**
Cooking time: **10 Min**
No. Of Servings: **3 Bowls**
Fridge Life: **1 Day**

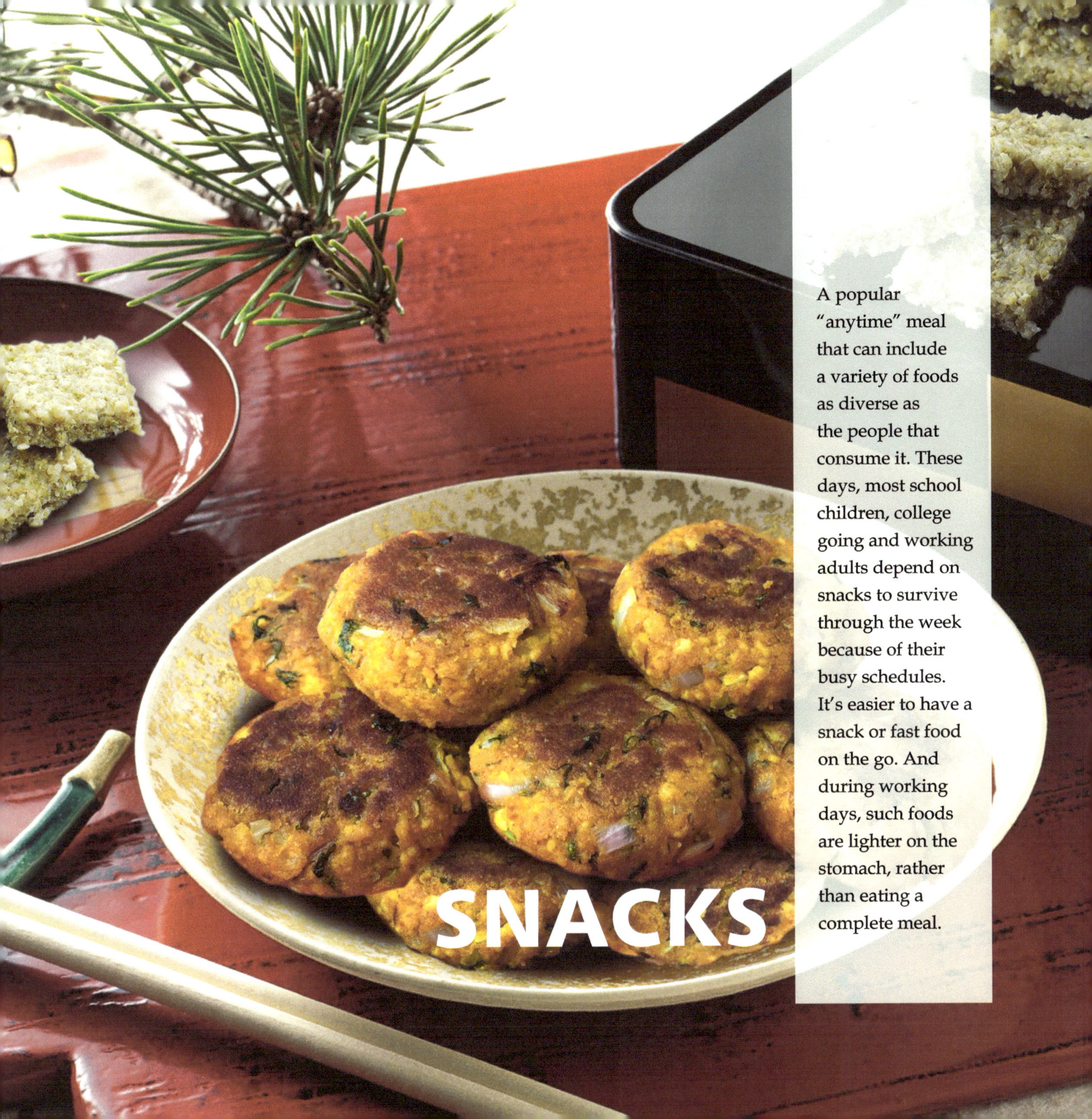

SNACKS

A popular "anytime" meal that can include a variety of foods as diverse as the people that consume it. These days, most school children, college going and working adults depend on snacks to survive through the week because of their busy schedules. It's easier to have a snack or fast food on the go. And during working days, such foods are lighter on the stomach, rather than eating a complete meal.

BUCKWHEAT (KUTTU) DHOKLA

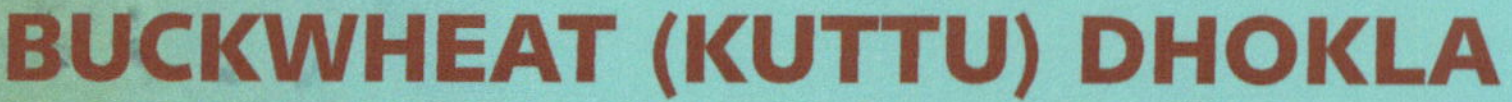

Buckwheat dhoklas are easy to make and can be had as mono meals, breakfast or anytime healthy snacks. Dhokla is a form of fermented batter made of rice or pulses. Despite the name, buckwheat is not related to wheat, as it is not a grass. It is often referred to as a pseudo cereal like amaranth and quinoa. Buckwheat is considered energizing and nutritious, and can be served as an alternative to rice or made into porridge. This dish tastes much better when eaten fresh.

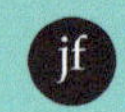

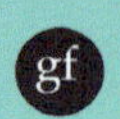

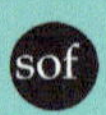

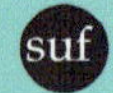

Ingredients

1. Kuttu *(Buckwheat)* (½ Cup)
2. Dairy-free Curd* (½ Cup)
3. Ginger-Chili Paste (1 Tsp. / Optional)
4. Roasted Cumin Powder (1/4 Tsp)
5. Roasted Peanuts, Semi-Crushed (1 Tbsp)
6. Rock Salt Or Unprocessed Sea Salt (1 Tbsp)
7. Cold-Pressed Oil (Few drops For Greasing)

Method

- Take a bowl and add kuttu as well as curd. Mix well. No need to add water.
- Leave it covered for minimum of 30 minutes and maximum of 6 hours. This will soften up the kuttu.
- Add 1 tsp. ginger chilies paste, 1/4 tsp. of roasted cumin powder, 1 tbsp of roasted semi-crushed peanuts and 1/2 tsp rock salt or unprocessed sea salt. Mix the ingredients well.
- Lightly grease the pan with cold pressed oil.
- Pour the mixture on the dish.
- Steam the dhokla in a steamer.
- Steam for 12-15min. The kuttu will be soft and puffy.
- With a knife, cut it into pieces. Let it cool for 2 minutes.
- Scoop the pieces with a flat spoon.
- Ready to serve. Enjoy!

* ***For dairy-free curd recipe,*** *refer to* ***Dairy Alternatives*** *by Dr Rupa Shah available on amazon.in and healthrevolution.in.*

BRIEF

Preparation (Soaking) Time: **30 Min-6 Hours**
Cooking Time: **15 Minutes**
No Of Servings: **1 Cup**
Fridge Life: **1 Day**

SPLIT CHAWLI DAAL (LOBIA) DHOKLA

Split-chili dhokla is made of black-eyed beans and is also known as *lobia*. It is very easy to make and a nutritious recipe. This dhokla is delicious, protein-rich and very light. Split-chili is rich with B-complex, protein, zinc, calcium and iron. It can be used as mono meals or for breakfast or an anytime-healthy snack.

jf sof gf nf suf

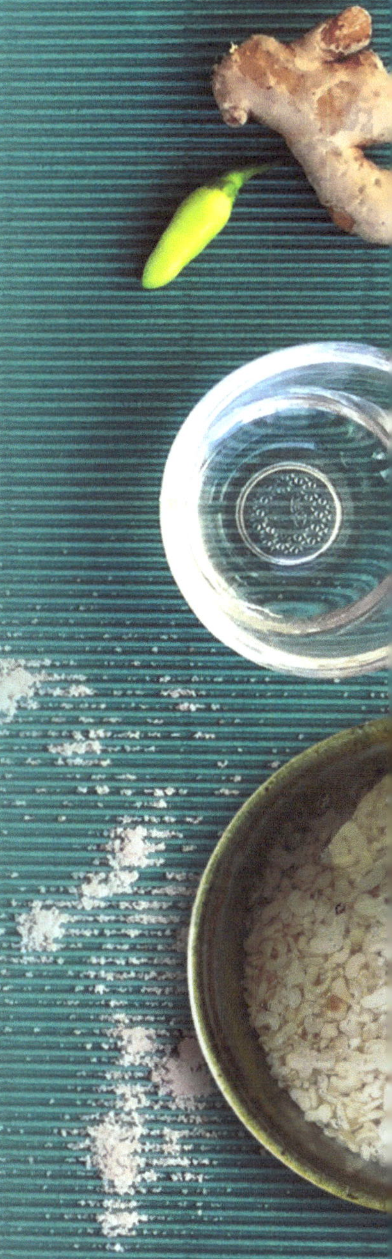

Ingredients

1. Split Chawli Daal *(Black-Eyed Bean)* as available in the market (1/2 Cup)
2. Water (1/2 Cup)
3. Ginger-Chili Paste (1 Tsp. / Optional)
4. Rock Salt Or Unprocessed Sea Salt (½ Tsp)
5. Cold-Pressed Oil (Few drops For Greasing)

Method

- Wash Split Chawli Daal well.
- Take a bowl and add Split Chawli Daal and water. Leave it covered for minimum of 6 hours and maximum of 8 hours. This will soften up split chili daal. Drain the water.
- Take ½ cup of water and blend this daal well. A stone grinder is also suitable.
- Add 1 Tsp. ginger-chili paste and ½ Tsp rock salt or unprocessed sea salt to the blended batter. Mix well.
- Take a dhokla dish and grease it lightly with cold pressed oil. Pour the mixture on the dish.
- Steam the chili daal mix in a dhokla steamer for 12-15min. The mixture will be will be soft and puffy.
- With a knife, cut it into pieces. Let it cool.
- Ready to serve. Enjoy!

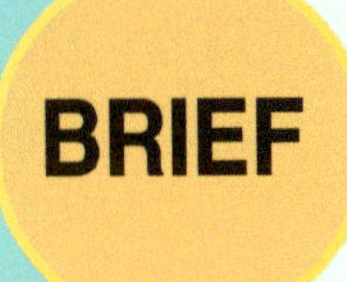

Preparation (Soaking)
Time: **6-8 Hours**
Cooking Time: **15 Min**
No. Of Servings: **1 Bowl**
Fridge Life: **1 Day**

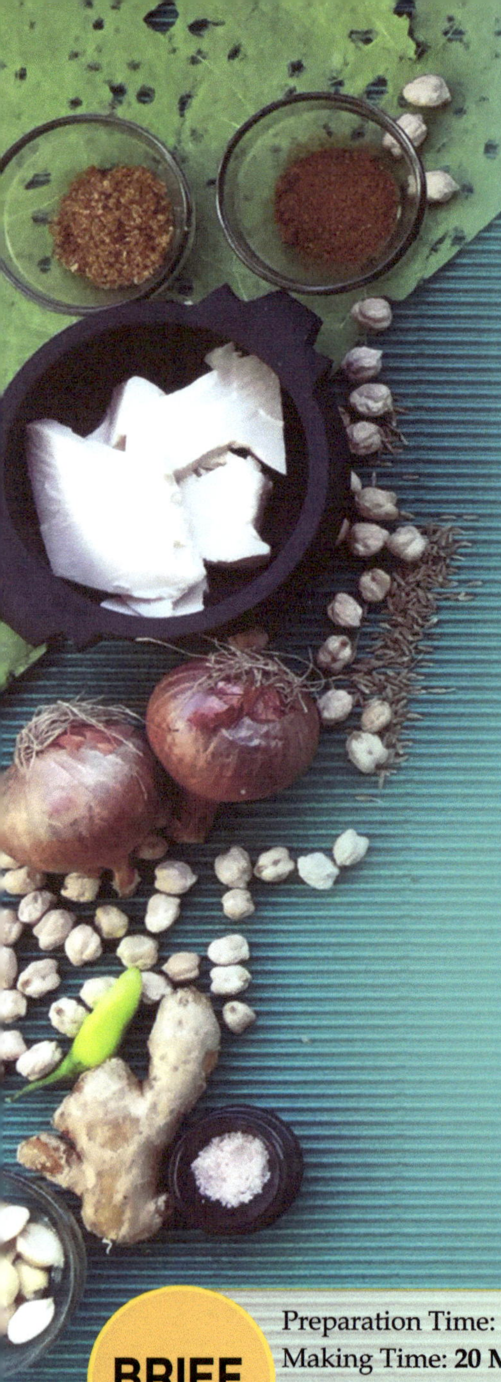

TOFU CUTLET

Tofu cutlet is a great snack. It can be had for breakfast as well. Add chickpeas to the mix and you have a power-packed calcium-rich meal as well.

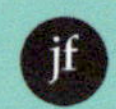 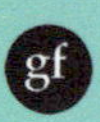 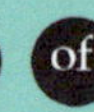 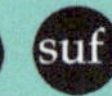

Ingredients

1. Tofu (200gm / Homemade preferred. Alternatively, buy readymade, firm variety)
2. Chickpeas, Cooked Until Soft (1 Cup)
3. Ginger-Chili Paste (1Tbsp/ Optional)
4. Rock or Sea Salt (1-1½ Tsp)
5. Roasted Cumin Powder (1 Tsp)
6. Fresh Coriander Leaves (2 Tbsp/ Finely Chopped)
7. Garam Masala/ Chat Masala (2 Tsp/ Optional)
8. Onion (1/ Finely Chopped/ Optional)
9. Roasted Peanut Powder (4 Tbsp)

Method

- Mash boiled chickpeas with a masher.
- Mix all the ingredients except peanut powder.
- Make round patty or whatever shape you like.
- Makes about 10 pieces. Roll these in peanut powder.
- Either bake in an oven or light roast on a pan.
- Serve hot with any chutney of your choice.

Tip: **No oil is required to bake as some oil will release from the peanuts.**

BRIEF

Preparation Time: **10 Min**
Making Time: **20 Min**
No. Of Servings: **10 Pc (Approx.)**
Fridge Life: **1 Day**

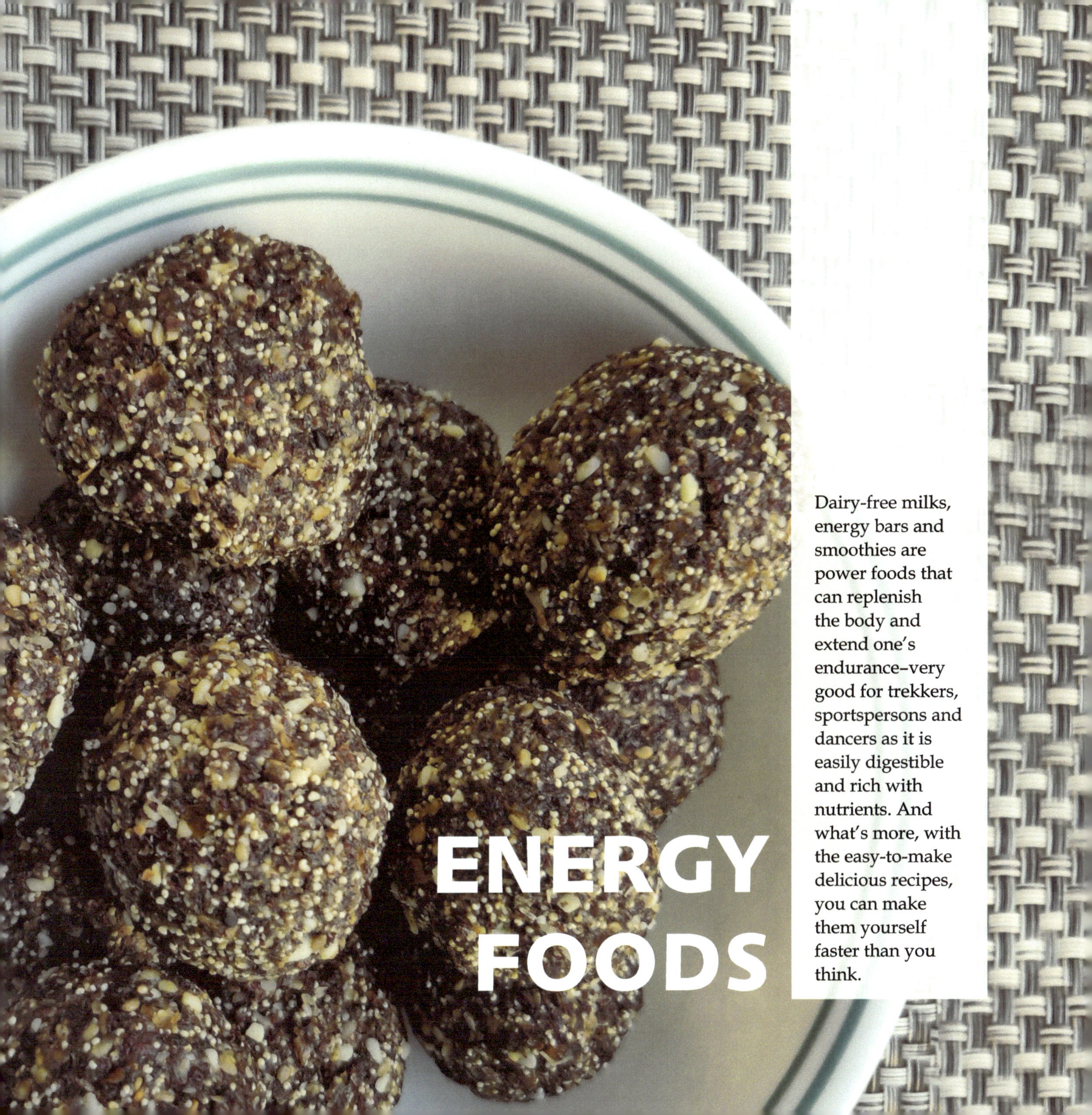

ENERGY FOODS

Dairy-free milks, energy bars and smoothies are power foods that can replenish the body and extend one's endurance–very good for trekkers, sportspersons and dancers as it is easily digestible and rich with nutrients. And what's more, with the easy-to-make delicious recipes, you can make them yourself faster than you think.

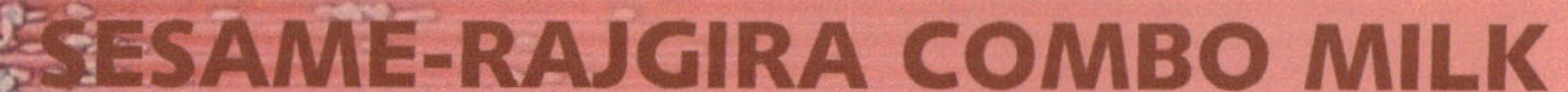

SESAME-RAJGIRA COMBO MILK

White Sesame-Rajgira *(Amaranth)* combo milk makes a rich and creamy beverage. Amaranth or rajgira means "immortal" or "everlasting" in Greek, possibly because it contains a high amount of calcium. It is also high in iron, magnesium, phosphorus, potassium and it is the only grain (actually a seed) which contains Vitamin C. Rajgira also reduces one's risk of osteoporosis, as it has twice the amount of calcium as dairy milk. This dairy-free milk will retain the flavour of sesame seeds, but can still be neutral tasting when you add cinnamon, dates and other flavors. Can be used for ice-cream as well.

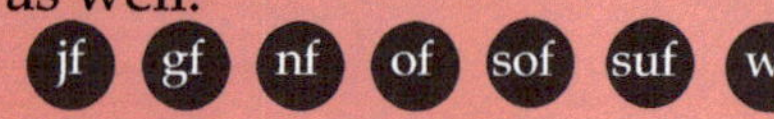

Ingredients

1. Raw White Sesame Seeds (1/2 Cup)
2. Roasted Puffed Rajigira (Amaranth) (1/2 Cup)
3. Fresh Water (2 cups/ Can also use coconut water for sweetness and electrolytes)
4. Natural Sweetener (Optional)
5. Cardamom, Vanilla Stick or Cocoa Powder for flavour (Optional)
6. Salt (A Pinch/ Optional)

Method

- Soak sesame seeds in ½ cup water for 6 to 8 hours.
- After 8 hours, drain the water.
- In a blender, add sesame seeds and roasted puffed rajgira with water. Blend well.

Tip 1: ***This is whole milk.*** *If you strain it, the milk is not whole food anymore, as the fibres and nutrients have been removed. More water can be added if you prefer thinner milk.*

Tip 2: You can add a pinch of salt, and a natural sweetener. Other flavourings options are cardamom, natural vanilla stick or cocoa powder.

BRIEF

Preparation (Soaking)
Time: **8 Hours**
Blending Time: **5 Min**
No. Of Servings: **1 Glass**
Fridge Life: **1 Day**
Note: Fresh milk tastes much better

NUTS & SEEDS BAR

This no-bake energy bar is simple and satisfying recipe that you just can't stop eating. You can make a number of combinations. These bars get their sweetness from dates, which also act as the glue that holds other ingredients together. Also, these quick-make bars are great for snacking when you're short on time.

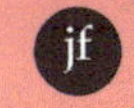 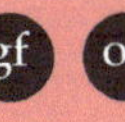 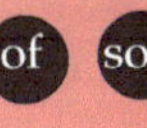 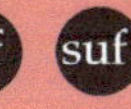 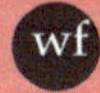

Ingredients

1. Roasted Roughly Chopped Almonds (½ Cup/ Unsalted)
2. Roasted Pistachios (¼ Cup Unsalted)
3. Walnuts (¼ Cup/ Unsalted)
4. Sunflower Seeds (1 Tbsp)
5. Roasted Sesame Seeds Black/ White (1 Tbsp Unsalted)
6. Flax Seeds (1 Tbsp)
7. Watermelon seeds (1 Tbsp)
8. Pumpkin seeds (1 Tbsp)
9. Dry coconut (2 Tbsp)
10. Raisins (2 Tbsp)
11. Dry, Deseeded Soft Dates (1/2-1 Cup-As Per Taste)
12. Dry deseeded Apricots (2Tbsp)
13. Coconut Palm Jaggery Paste (4Tbsp)
14. Peanut Butter (¼ Cup)
15. Cinnamon Powder (Pinch)
16. Salt (Pinch)

Method

- Blend the nuts and seeds in a food processor by pulsing method for just a minute. This way nuts and seeds are not fully crushed, but semi-crushed.
- Add raisins, dates and apricots. Pulse again.
- Add jaggery and peanut butter. Blend again and let the mixture get a bit sticky.
- Lay this mixture on a flat surface dish or pan.
- Press well. Allow it to firm up in a refrigerator for about an hour.
- Cut into pieces.

BRIEF

Preparation time: **15 Min**
Making Time: **10 Min**
No Of Pc: **30 Pc (Approx.)**
Fridge Life: **Not Required**
Note: Can keep outside for a month

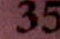

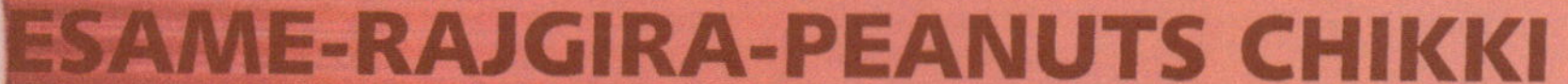

SESAME-RAJGIRA-PEANUTS CHIKKI

These combo-chikkis (brittle sweets) or single nut and seed chikkis are available at most kirana shops, and Lonavala is also best known for its chikkis. However, those are coated with corn syrup or sugar. Here is some good news–it's easy to make these at home by yourself and also healthier. Read on to know how.

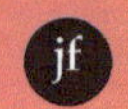

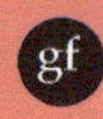

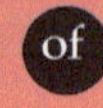

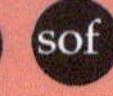

Ingredients

1. Rajgira (*Amaranth*) Puffs (3 Cups)
2. Roasted Peanuts (2 Tbsp/Semi-Crushed)
3. Roasted White Sesame Seeds (2 Tbsp)
4. Jaggery (1-2 Cup/s-As Per Taste)
5. Water (1 Tbsp)

Method

- In a pan, take 1 Tbsp water. Heat it a bit and add jaggery until it melts and is cooked. Constantly stir the jaggery for about 2 minutes until can see the jaggery foaming. Turn off the stove.
- Add rajgira puffs, semi-crushed peanuts and roasted sesame seeds.
- Stir the mix well.
- Keep a flat dish ready on the side. Spread this mixture on the steel flat dish and press a bit. With knife, make lines to cut the pieces of chikki. Alternatively, one can wet hands with a bit of water and roll laddoos (balls) out of this mixture. Cool in for 3 hours outside and cut it into pieces.
- Store it in cool, dry, airtight container.

Note: Peanuts and sesame seeds can be dry-roasted separately for 3 minutes each, before-hand.

BRIEF

Preparation Time: **15 Min**
Cooking Time: **5 Min**
No. Of Pc: **15**
Fridge Life: **Not Required**
Note: **Can keep outside for a month**

BLACK TIL LADDOO

COURTESY: PARUL MEHTA

Black til (sesame) is valued for its oil. It contains even more calcium than its white counterpart. You can include these nutrient-rich seeds in your cereals, rice, noodles or mix them with yoghurt or smoothie for a rich nutty flavor. These laddoos or balls are yummy tasting and very nutritious and filling especially during the winter.

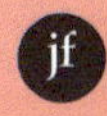

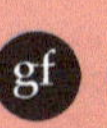

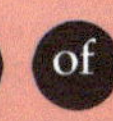

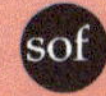

Ingredients

1. Black Til or Black Sesame Seeds (500g)
2. Raw Peanuts (250g Cup)
3. Natural Or Organic Jaggery (400gm)

Method

- Roast peanuts, remove the skin and set aside.
- Roast til.
- In a dry blender, blend peanuts into fine powder.
- Blend sesame seeds and make into fine powder.
- Mix all with jaggery powder and blend in dry blender again till all jaggery mixes well and looks like dough.
- Knead for about 2 minutes till the dough seems well blended.
- From the dough, pull out small portions and make small laddoos (balls) and serve.
- Store in a dry container.

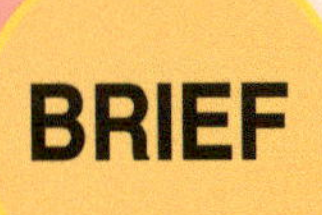

Preparation Time: **5 Min**
Cooking Time: **10 Min**
No. Of Pc: **20 Balls (Approx.)**
Fridge Life: Not Required
Note: **Can keep outside for a month**

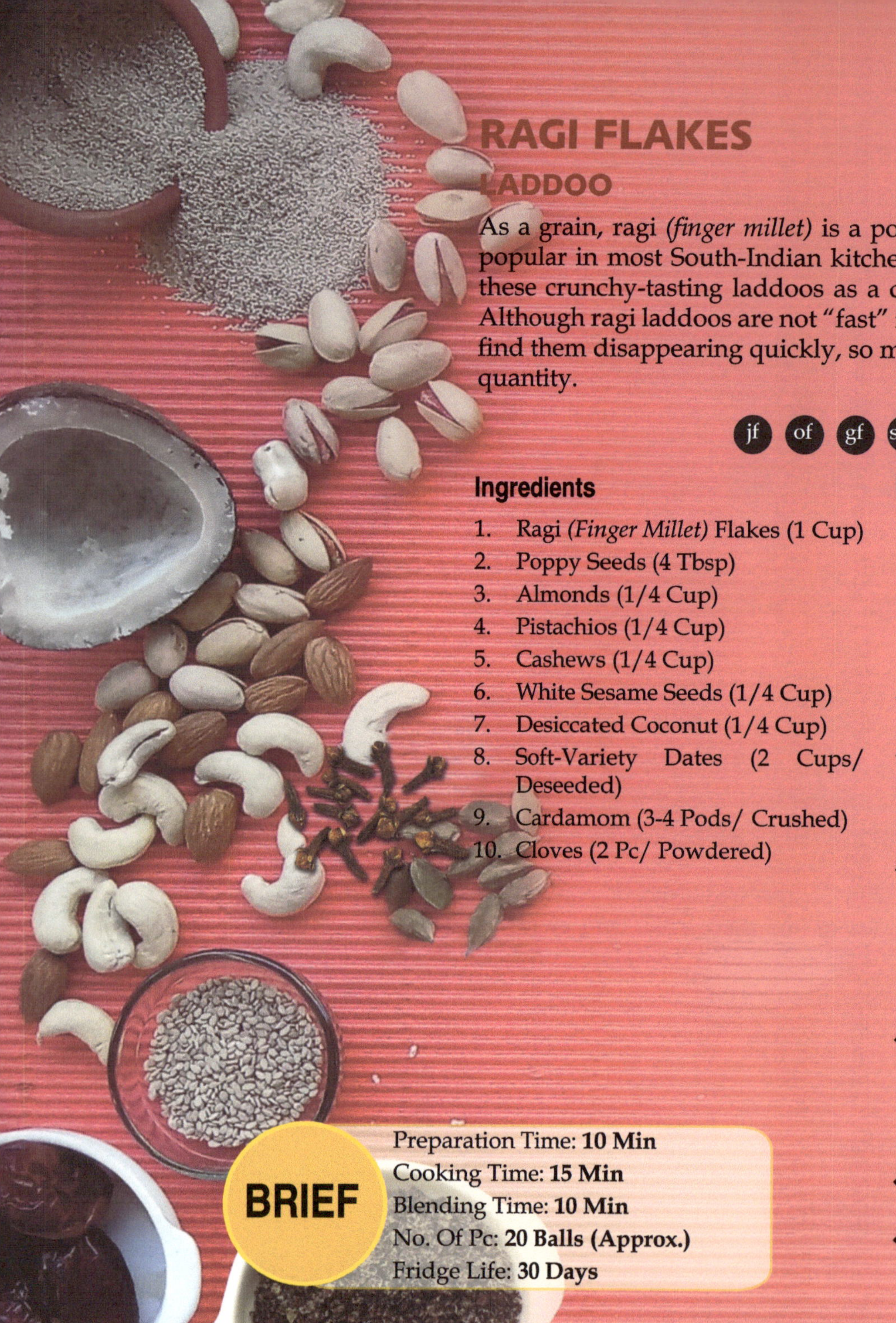

RAGI FLAKES
LADDOO

As a grain, ragi *(finger millet)* is a powerhouse of nutrition and is very popular in most South-Indian kitchens. You can tempt your kids with these crunchy-tasting laddoos as a change from usual routine snacks. Although ragi laddoos are not "fast" food, they are so tasty that you will find them disappearing quickly, so make sure you have made sufficient quantity.

jf of gf sof suf wf

Ingredients

1. Ragi *(Finger Millet)* Flakes (1 Cup)
2. Poppy Seeds (4 Tbsp)
3. Almonds (1/4 Cup)
4. Pistachios (1/4 Cup)
5. Cashews (1/4 Cup)
6. White Sesame Seeds (1/4 Cup)
7. Desiccated Coconut (1/4 Cup)
8. Soft-Variety Dates (2 Cups/ Deseeded)
9. Cardamom (3-4 Pods/ Crushed)
10. Cloves (2 Pc/ Powdered)

Method

- Chop the dates roughly and using a food processor or grinder, pulse the dates in small batches. This will make small bits and save you the time and effort of individually chopping the dates.
- Make the cardamom and clove into fine powder.
- In a wok, dry roast the almonds and cashews. Keep aside. Repeat process with sesame and poppy seeds.
- In the processor, add the roasted cashews and pulse briefly for semi-crushed texture. Add ragi flakes, and roasted sesame and poppy seeds, pistachios and dry coconut flakes. Pulse again.
- Add the dates and pulse until the dates have blended well the with the mixture. Pulse well for a few minutes. Mixture is ready to be rolled out into balls.
- Pinch out small portions from the mix and roll into balls.
- Store in an air-tight container.

BRIEF

Preparation Time: **10 Min**
Cooking Time: **15 Min**
Blending Time: **10 Min**
No. Of Pc: **20 Balls (Approx.)**
Fridge Life: **30 Days**

RADISH LEAVES SMOOTHIE

Radish leaves may not be the first idea that comes to mind when you are making a smoothie, but radish leaves are a super source of calcium, iron, magnesium, folate, vitamins A, C, K and many other nutrients. This thick beverage is delicious and is a super way to give your body a healthy boost.

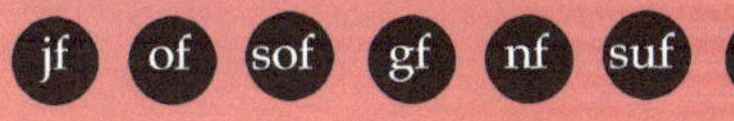

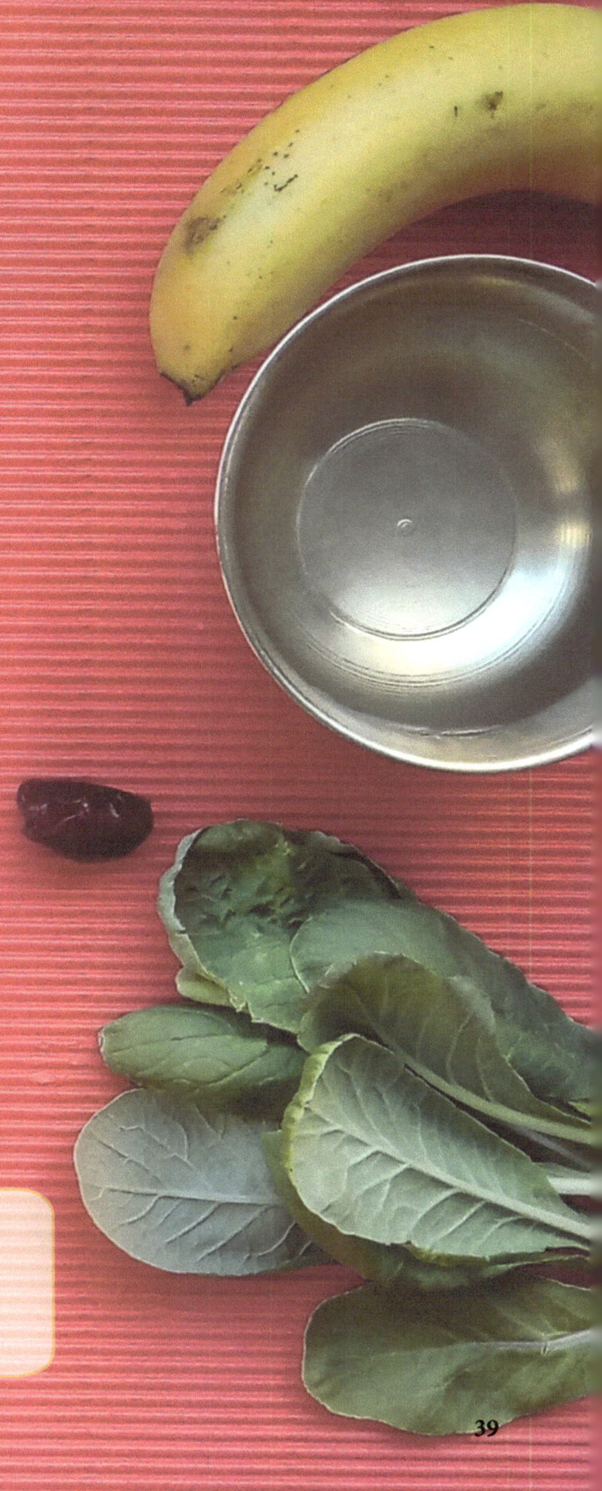

Ingredients

1. Ripe Banana (1 Pc/ or Use Frozen Banana for Chilled Taste)
2. Raw Radish Leaves (10) (Washed Well)
3. Fresh Water (1 Glass)
4. Deseeded Dates (1 Pc/ Optional)

Method

- Blend all of ingredients for 2 minutes.
- Serve in a nice glass.

Note: *Most of us have been throwing away radish greens for years. Unfortunately, we have thrown away a significant source of calcium, iron, magnesium and folate, as well as vitamins A, C, K and other nutrients. Not only are radish greens edible, the leaves are the most nutritious part of the plant.*

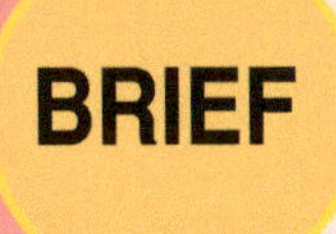

Preparation Time: **5 Min**
Making Time: **5 Min**
No. of Servings: **1 Glass**
Fridge Life: **1 Day**

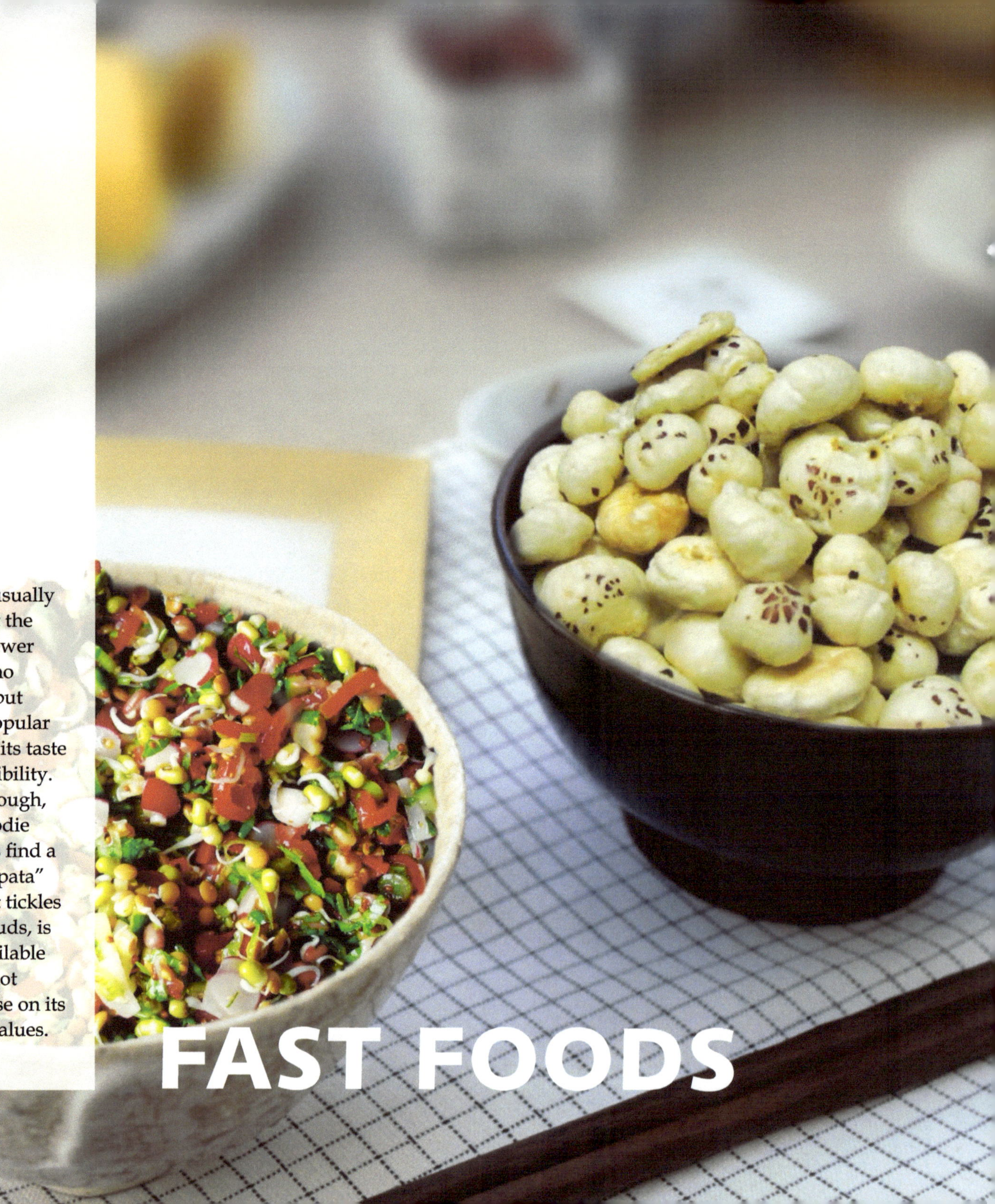

Fast food usually means that the food has fewer or almost no nutrients, but globally popular because of its taste and accessibility. In India though, a smart foodie can always find a local "chatpata" option that tickles the taste-buds, is locally available and does not compromise on its nutrition values.

FAST FOODS

SPROUT BHEL

Bhel (a popular Indian street-food that is a type of Rice Puff Salad) is sure to be an all-time favourite *chatpata* snack with the family. This version of raw sprout salad bhel will boost your energy and protein requirements when you sometimes feel like munching on a snack. The combination of moong and math sprouts will provide you with calcium, vitamins and fibre, and you can munch this without worrying about weight gain.

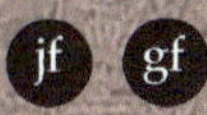

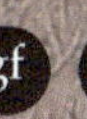

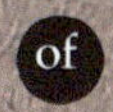

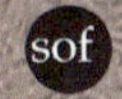

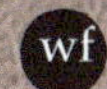

Ingredients

1. Puffed Rice (3 Cups)
2. Mung Sprouts (1 Tbsp)
3. Math Sprouts (1 Tbsp. / Turkish Gram or Moth Bean)
4. Sprouted Kulith or *Horse Gram* (1 Tbsp)
5. Chopped Onion (1/2/ Optional)
6. Chopped Tomato (1 Pc)
7. Boiled Potato (1/2 /Chopped/ Optional)
8. Roasted Peanuts (No. 12-15)
9. Lemon Juice (2 Tsp) Or Raw Mango (Chopped/ 1 Tbsp)
10. Chaat Masala as Per Taste
11. 1 Green Chili (Finely Chopped/ Optional)
12. Pomegranate seeds (2 Tbsp/ Optional)
13. Coriander Leaves (Freshly chopped/ For Garnishing)
14. Rock Salt To Taste

Method

- In a bowl, mix puffed rice, all the sprouts, onion, tomato, potato and peanuts.
- Squeeze lemon juice, add chaat masala, salt, green chili, and mix again.
- Garnish with coriander and serve.

Tip: ***Add Coriander- Mint Chutney & Date Chutney to perk up the recipe.***

BRIEF

Preparation Time: **15 Min**
Cooking Time: **20 Min**
No. Of Servings: **4 Cups**
Fridge Life: **1 Day**

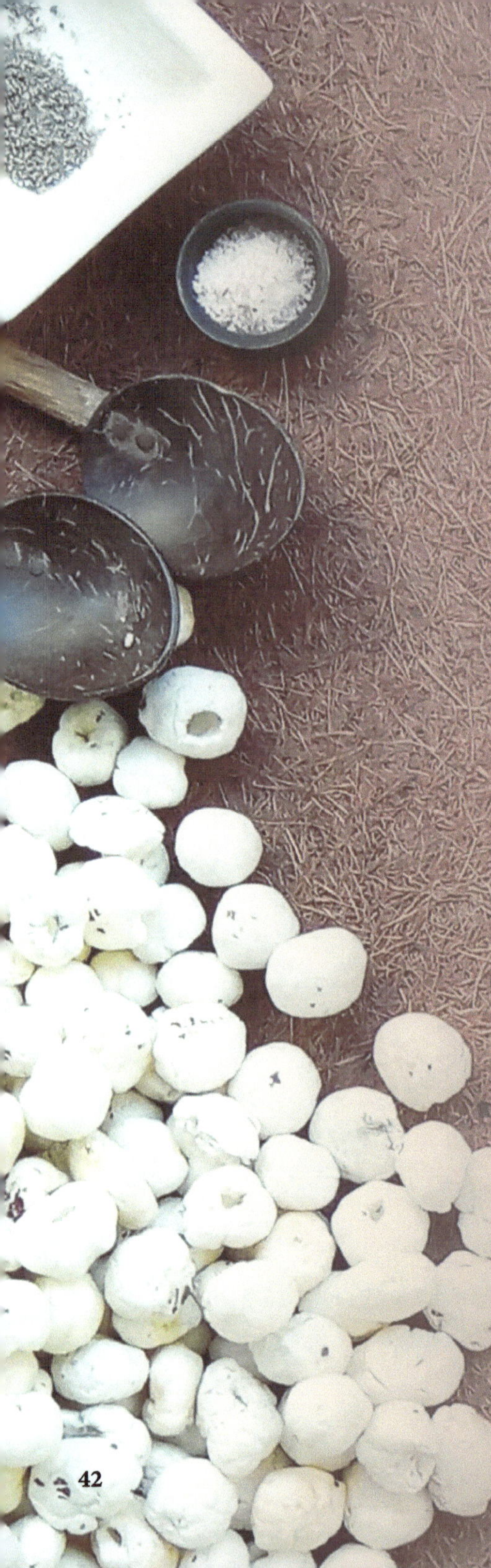

ROASTED WATER LILY
(PHOOL MAKHANA) SEEDS

Also called fox nuts, roasted water-lily seeds are a popular desi version of popcorn. It is rich in calcium, phosphorus, zinc and iron. They may be almost tasteless by themselves, but when tempered with the right condiments and spices, they turn into crunchy, yummy and any-time snack. It is readily available in the market as makhana, but one can also make it at home.

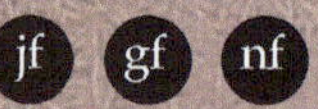

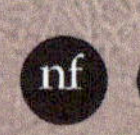

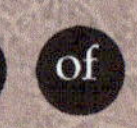

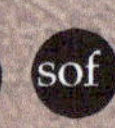

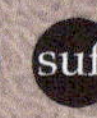

Ingredients

1. Makhanas Or *Water Lily Seeds* (3 Cup)
2. Black Pepper (1 Tsp)
3. Rock Salt To Taste

Method

- Heat a pan on a low flame for 5 minutes
- Roast the makhanas on the pan for about 14-15 minutes or until they become crunchy from outside.
- Add rock salt and black pepper powder for taste. Or eat as it is.

***Tip:* You can alternatively replace black pepper with turmeric powder or chat masala.**

Trivia: *Makhanas come from a plant called Euryale Fox which grows in the stagnant water of wetlands or ponds in Bihar, Manipur in India, Korea, Japan and parts of Russia. Moreover, they have been used in Chinese medicine for 3,000 years and have their place in Ayurveda as well.*

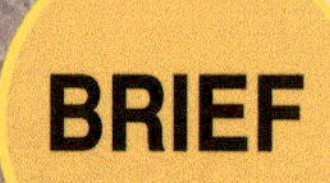

Preparation Time: **15 Min**
Cooking Time: **10 Min**
No. Of Servings: **4 Cups**
Fridge Life: **3 Days**

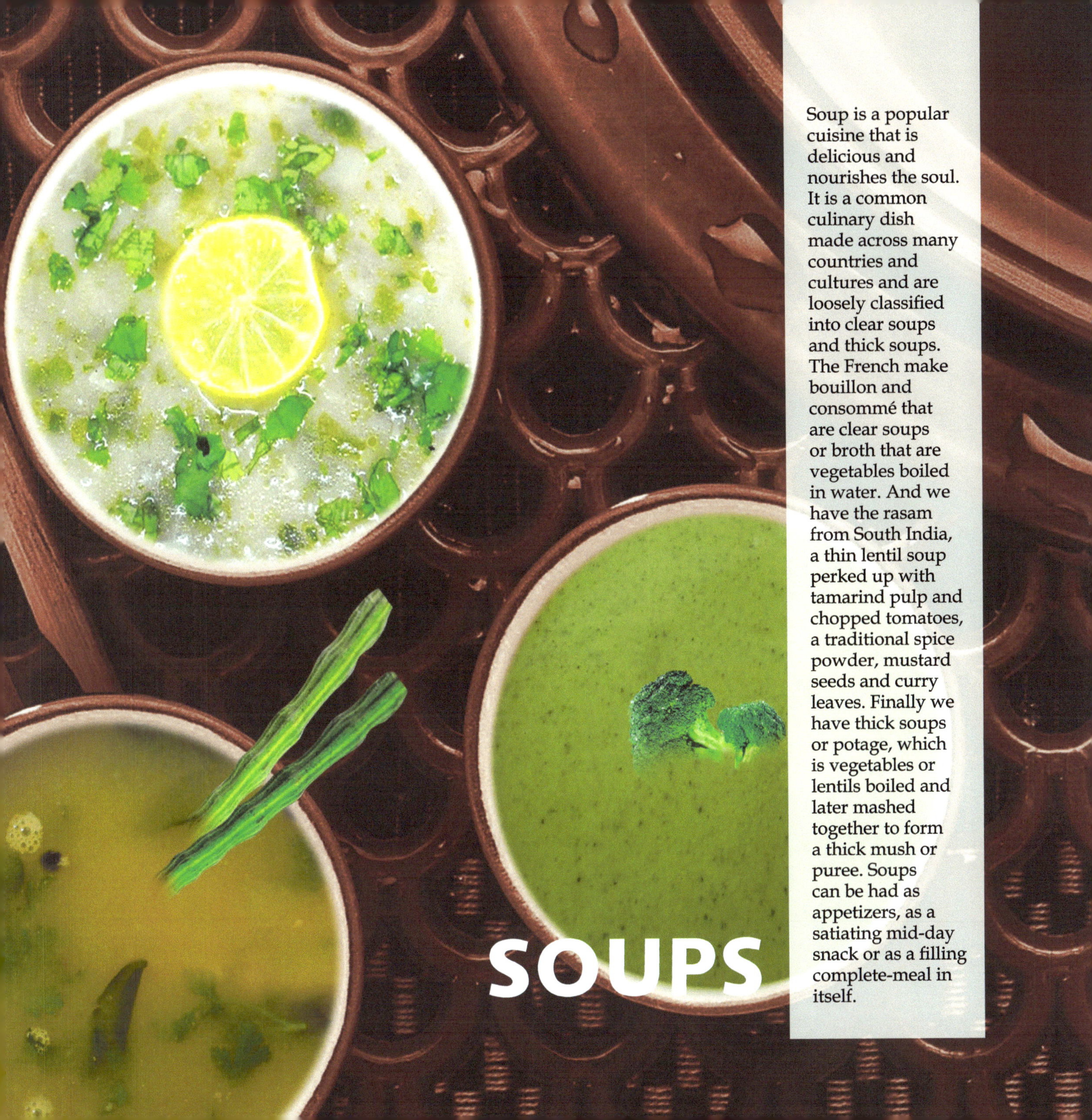

SOUPS

Soup is a popular cuisine that is delicious and nourishes the soul. It is a common culinary dish made across many countries and cultures and are loosely classified into clear soups and thick soups. The French make bouillon and consommé that are clear soups or broth that are vegetables boiled in water. And we have the rasam from South India, a thin lentil soup perked up with tamarind pulp and chopped tomatoes, a traditional spice powder, mustard seeds and curry leaves. Finally we have thick soups or potage, which is vegetables or lentils boiled and later mashed together to form a thick mush or puree. Soups can be had as appetizers, as a satiating mid-day snack or as a filling complete-meal in itself.

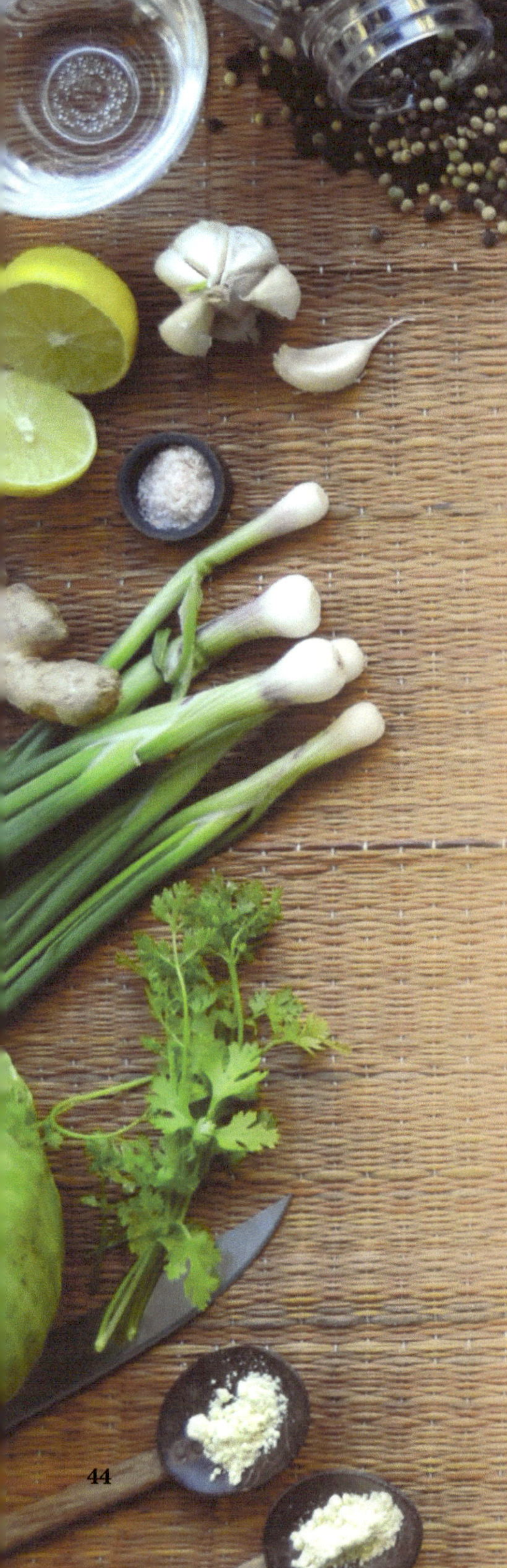

LIME CORIANDER SOUP

This light and refreshing soup is rich with Vitamin C and a good resource to boost your natural immunity. It will also help relieve cough and cold. Health benefits apart, this soup is simple and makes a yummy piping hot meal during the monsoons and through winters alike. It is one of our favourite soups because of its fragrance, and it's a great appetizer as well.

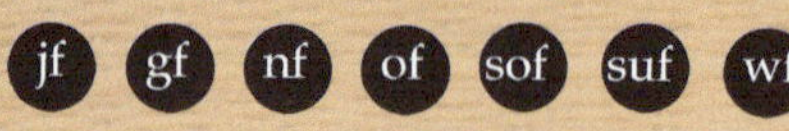

Ingredients

1. Fresh Lime Juice (2 Tbsp)
2. Freshly Chopped Coriander Leaves (2 Tbsp) With Chopped Stems Kept Separately
3. Spring Onions (Chopped With Green Shoots/1 Bulb/ Optional)
4. Garlic Crushed (1 Small Clove/ Optional)
5. Crushed Ginger (1 Small Pc/ Optional)
6. Gram Flour (2 Tbsp)
7. Vegetable Stock (4 Cups) or drinking water
8. Chopped Cabbage (¼ Cup)
9. Freshly Crushed Black Peppercorns to Taste
10. Rock Salt To Taste

Method

- In a pan, dry roast onion, garlic and ginger for 2 minutes.
- Add gram flour and dry roast the flour till you can smell the aroma.
- Add vegetable stock water, coriander stems and chopped cabbage. Cook a bit and bring it to boil.
- Add crushed peppercorns and chopped coriander leaves. Continue to boil.
- Add rock salt as per taste. Turn off the stove.
- Add lime juice. Do not boil after lime juice is added.
- Cover for 2 minutes.
- The soup is ready to serve.

Note: ***For Jain cooking, start directly from Step 2 by dry roasting the gram flour***

BRIEF

Preparation Time: **10 Min**
Cooking Time: **20 Min**
No. of Servings: **2 Bowls (Approx.)**
Fridge Life: **1 Day**

MORINGA-DRUMSTICK SOUP

Drumsticks as a vegetable are seed pods of Moringa Oleifera and are high in vitamin C. It is a good source of dietary fibre, potassium, magnesium, and manganese. Add drumstick leaves or moringa leaves and you have a power recipe as the leaves are highly nutritious, not only for their protein content— they are also packed with beta-carotene, vitamin C, calcium, potassium, and iron. Make sure to chew the leaves well to assimilate the maximum amount of nutrients. Now let's get to the Moringa-Drumstick soup recipe.

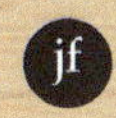

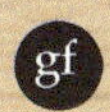

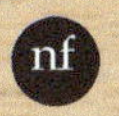

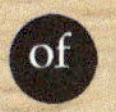

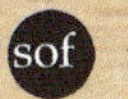

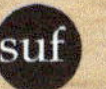

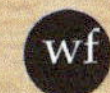

Ingredients

1. Moringa Leaves (Washed) (1/4 Cup)
2. Drumsticks (4 Sticks)
3. Water For Boiling (2 Cups)
4. Chopped Tomatoes (2 No's)
5. Cumin Seeds (1 Tsp)
6. Thin Watery Boiled Moong Dal (2 cup)
7. Curry Leaves
8. Fresh Coriander Leaves (Chopped)
9. Salt As Per Taste
10. Black Pepper Powder as Per Taste
11. Cinnamon (1 Pod)

Method

- Wash the moringa leaves and wipe them well.
- Wash the drumsticks thoroughly. Chop them into 2-inches long pieces.
- Boil moringa with drumsticks in 2 cups of water. The sticks should become soft. Scoop out the drumstick pulp with a spoon and discard the harder covers. This may take 10 minutes.
- Blend the pulp well and keep aside.
- In a pan, dry roast the cumin seeds for a minute.
- Add chopped tomatoes and cook a bit.
- Add the watery moong dal and cook a bit. Add left-over water from boiled drumstick pulp also.
- Add drumstick-moringa pulp, salt and black pepper powder.
- Boil for about 2 minutes.
- Garnish with cinnamon, curry leaves and coriander leaves.
- Serve hot.

Note: ***Leftover water can be used in the soup.***

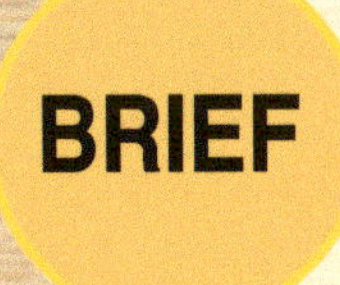

Preparation Time: **10 Min**
Cooking Time: **20 Min**
No. Of Servings: **2 Bowls (Approx.)**
Fridge Life: **1 Day**

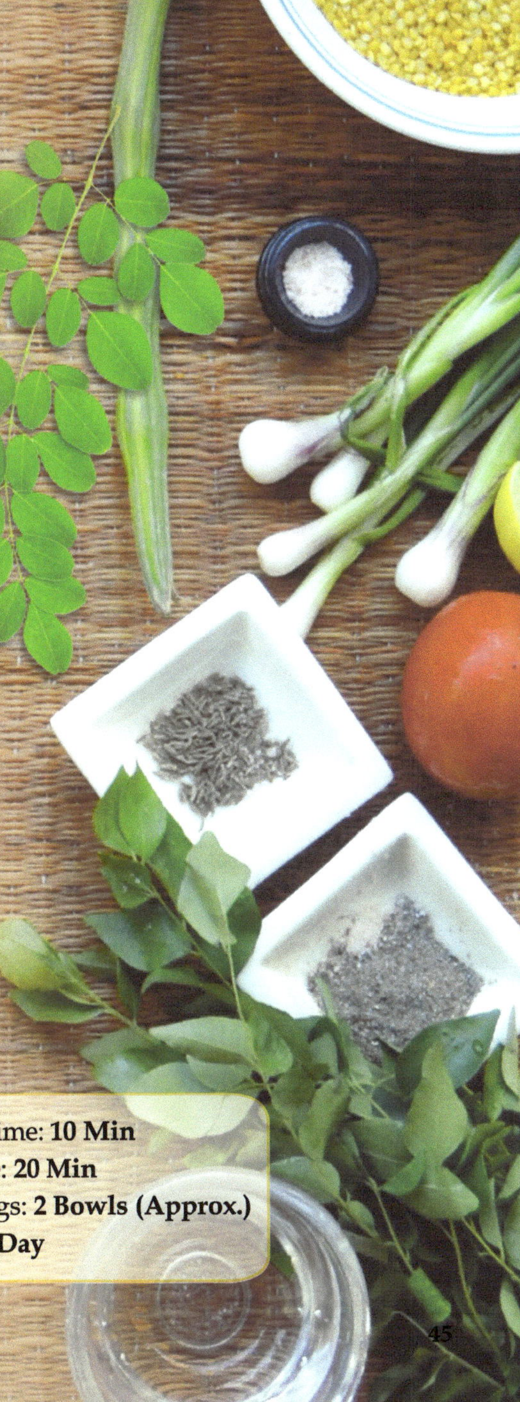

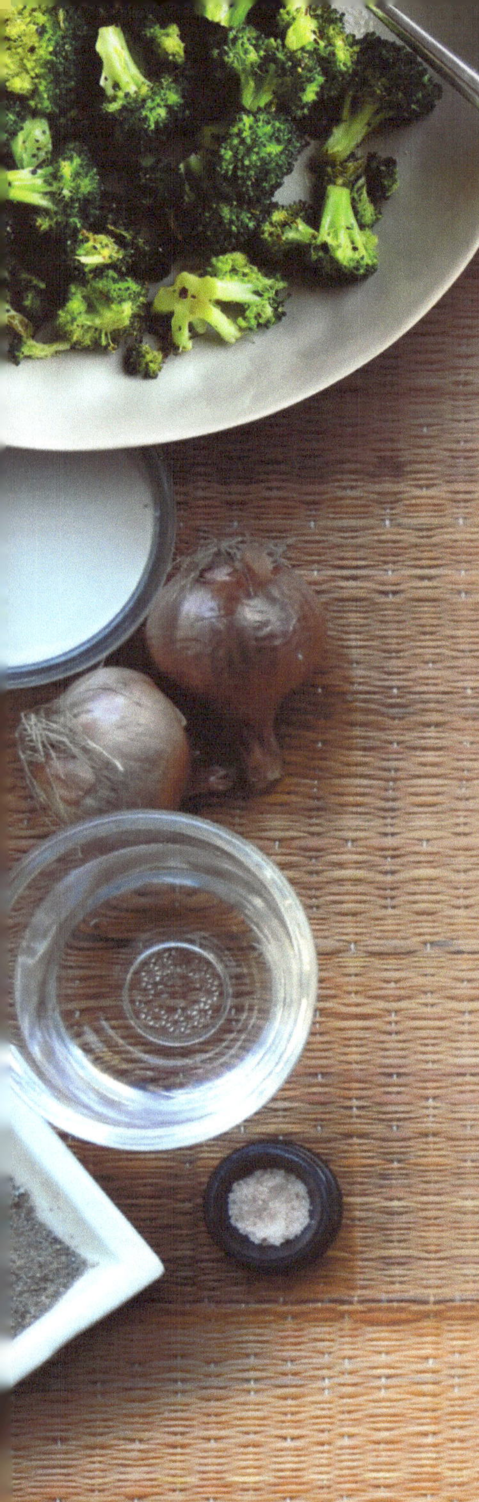

BROCCOLI SOUP

Broccoli is not the most loved vegetable in the house, but it makes an awesome soup. Try this recipe, as it makes a great accompaniment with a vegetable curry, pasta or a stir-fry or even assorted breads. It is simple, smooth and flavourful and makes a perfect starter to a dinner party.

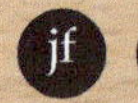

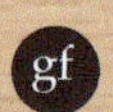

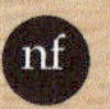

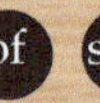

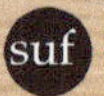

Ingredients

1. Broccoli (250gm/ Chopped In Large Pieces)
2. Onion (Chopped/ I Pc/ Optional)
3. Thick Coconut Milk* (½ Cup)
4. Black Pepper Powder or As Per Taste (½ Tsp)
5. Water (2 Cups for Blending)
6. Rock Salt or As Per Taste (½ Tsp)

Method

- Lightly steam broccoli and onions for about 5 minutes. Cool.
- Blend both to make puree.
- Pour puree in a pan. Add 1 cup water to make it thinner.
- Add salt and pepper.
- Boil this soup for 5 minutes.
- Add coconut milk and turn off the flame. Stir well.
- Soup is ready. Serve hot.

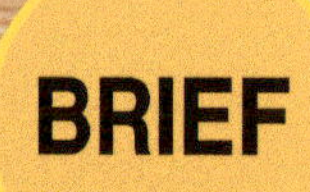

Preparation Time: **10 minutes**
Cooking Time: **20 Minutes**
No. Of Servings: **2 Bowls (Approx.)**
Fridge Life: **1 Day**

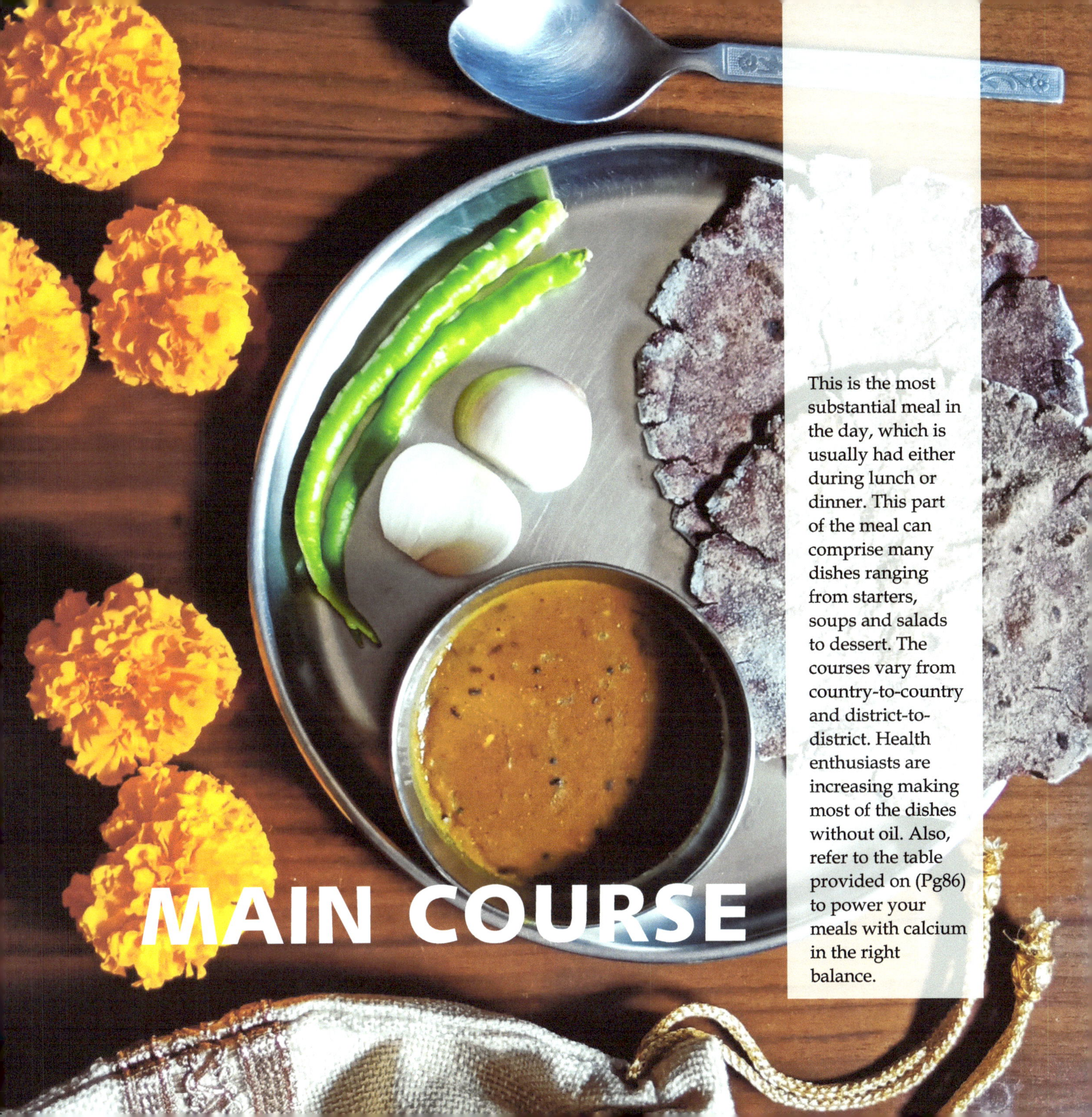

MAIN COURSE

This is the most substantial meal in the day, which is usually had either during lunch or dinner. This part of the meal can comprise many dishes ranging from starters, soups and salads to dessert. The courses vary from country-to-country and district-to-district. Health enthusiasts are increasing making most of the dishes without oil. Also, refer to the table provided on (Pg86) to power your meals with calcium in the right balance.

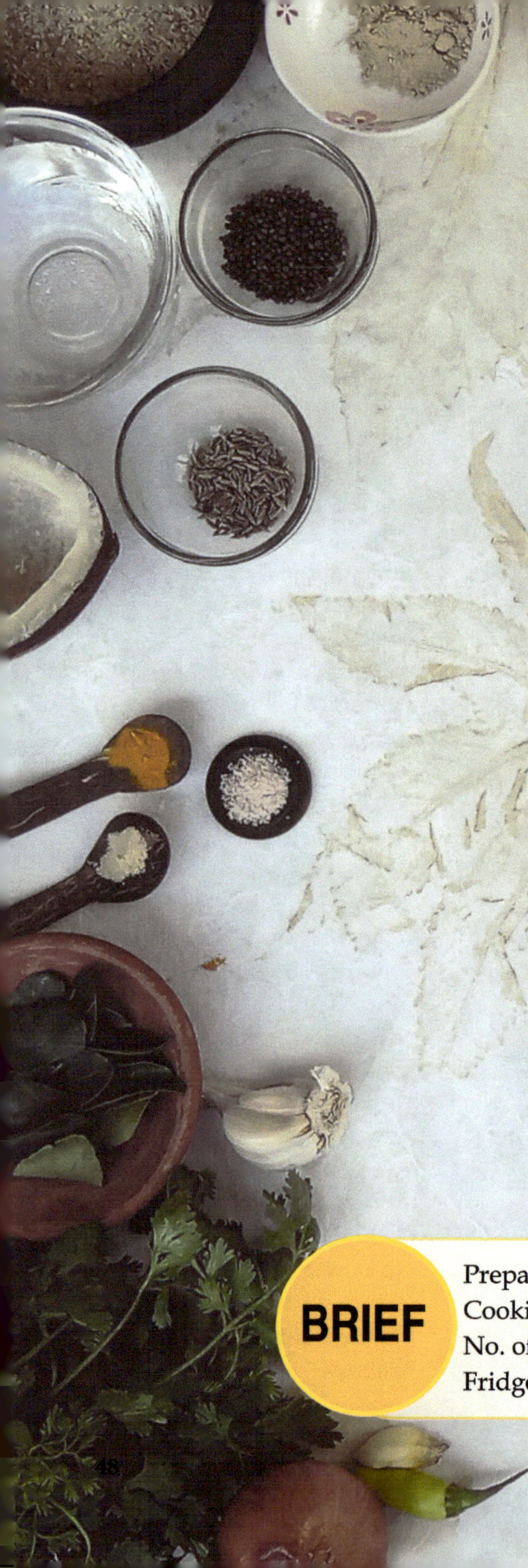

KULITH PITHLA

This Maharashtrian recipe is easy to prepare. *Kulith, kulthi* or Madras Gram are local names of Horse Gram, which was during early days fed to horses as it generates lots of energy, and that is how it got its name. It is a lesser type of bean and is known to generate heat in body, so, it is usually eaten in winter. It is a great comfort food that is loaded with power and is delicious, and healthy as well.

jf gf nf of sof suf wf

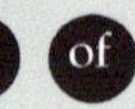

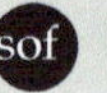

Ingredients

1. Kulith *(Horse Gram)* Flour (½ Cup)
2. Green Chilies (2 Pc)
3. Garlic Cloves (2 Pc/ Optional)
4. Onion (1 Medium size/ Chopped/ Optional)
5. Dry Coconut (¼ Cup)
6. Mustard Seeds (1 Tsp)
7. Cumin Seeds (Jeera/ 1 Tsp)
8. Turmeric Powder (1 Tsp)
9. Hing (Asafoetida/ Pinch)
10. Dried Kokum (2 Pc Or Amchur Powder (½ tsp.) Or Imli (*Tamarind*) Paste
11. Curry Leaves (Few)
12. Fresh Water (1 Cup + 3 Cups)
13. Coriander Leaves for Garnishing
14. Rock Salt as Per Taste

Method

- Dry roast coconut and cumin seeds in a pan, separately. Keep aside.
- Grind coconut and cumin seeds.
- Mix kulith flour in 1 cup of water well. Make sure there are no lumps.
- Dry roast green chilies and garlic in the pan.
- Add mustard seeds and dry roast the same. It will splutter soon.
- Add curry leaves, turmeric powder and hing. Gently stir for a few seconds.
- Add onions. Roast till it turns golden brown.
- Add coconut-cumin mixture and roast it for some time.
- Add 3 cups of water and bring it to a boil.
- Add kokum and salt as required.
- Add the kulith batter slowly and gently stir this while it is getting mixed.
- Cook the mixture for about 10 minutes while stirring often so that it does not stick to the pan.
- Garnish this dish with freshly chopped coriander leaves.
- Serve hot with rice *bhakri* or rice or roti.

BRIEF

Preparation Time: **15 Min**
Cooking Time: **20 Min**
No. of servings: **4 Cups**
Fridge Life: **1 Day**

CURRY LEAVES & CAULIFLOWER GREEN WHOLE WHEAT ROTI

Cauliflower greens are a very good source of nutrition, although we often discard the leaves. We recommend that you utilize them in your rotis. And fortify it with curry leaves and you have a complete meal in itself. You can use this roti as a wrap or as a burrito. How-so-ever you eat it, they are power-packed with nutrition without compromising on taste. We suggest you try this roti-wrap with the **Stir-Fry** recipe (**Pg56**) and **Basil-Pesto Sauce** (**Pg 75**).

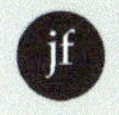

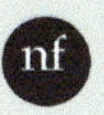

of
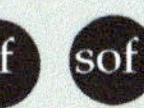

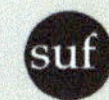

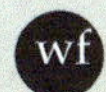

Ingredients

1. Whole Wheat Flour (2 Cups)
2. Curry Leaves (100gm)
3. Cauliflower Greens (100gm)
4. Salt to Taste
5. Fresh Water (As Required)

Method

- Wash curry leaves and cauliflower green leaves well.
- Now blend this, making it like thick paste. Add this paste to the whole wheat flour. Also add salt.
- Knead it well and make it into nice soft dough.
- Cover the dough with wet cloth for 2 hours. There will be natural fermentation of the dough as the dough will increase in size.
- Now make small balls and roll out roti and cook it on the tawa like any roti.
- Eat right away.

Tip: ***Can also use clean soft stems of leaves.***

Note: ***If you need to store, then store the rotis in a container at the bottom and cover it with cotton cloth and keep in an airtight container. They will remain fresh for up to 2 hours.***

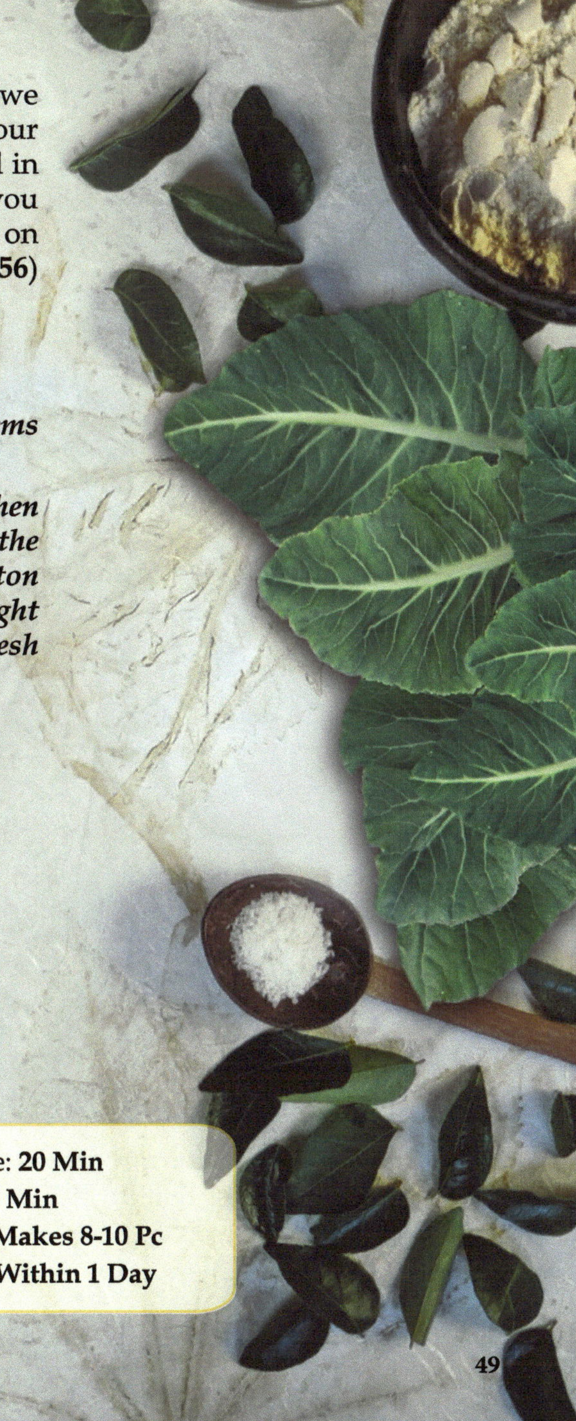

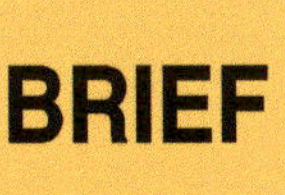

Preparation Time: **20 Min**
Cooking time: **10 Min**
No. of servings: **Makes 8-10 Pc**
Fridge Life: **Use Within 1 Day**

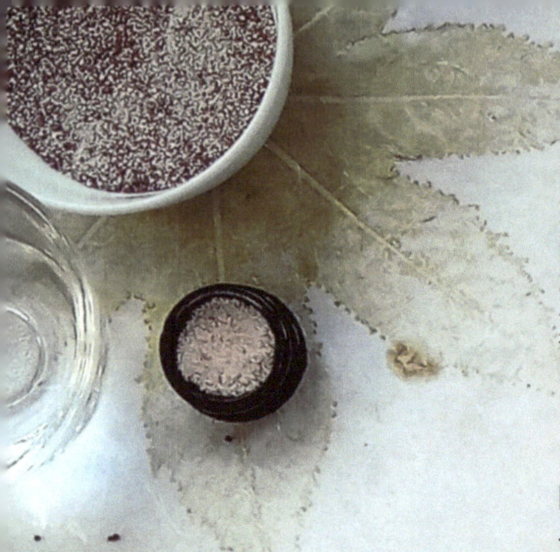

NACHANI (FINGER MILLET) ROTI

Nachani, also called *ragi* locally, or finger millets is a gluten-free shortbread is a much healthier alternative to its *atta* avatar common across most households. *Ragi* is a popular staple in Karnataka and as popular in Maharashtra as well. Roll them out thin and they taste even better with raita or chutney.

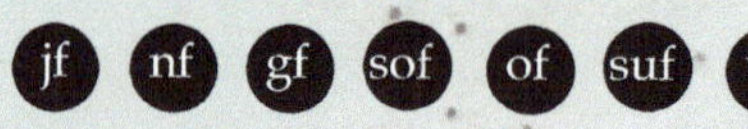

Ingredients

1. Nachani Flour *(Finger Millets)* (1 Cup)
2. Hot water For Kneading the Dough
3. Rock Salt to Taste

Method

- Put nachani flour in a bowl and pour hot water at the center.
- With a spatula, mix water gently in the flour.
- Let it cool a bit and add rock salt and knead the dough.
- Make balls from the dough. Rollout thick roti, one a time.
- On a tawa, dry roast the roti on both the sides just as it is done for roti. You may also cook it on the flame to let it puff up. However, we prefer to use a wire mesh to not let gas flame directly touch the roti. Do not use oil here.
- Serve hot with chutney or raita or any bhaji.

Tip: Try and replace calcium pills with a ragi kanji or porridge. This is a good way to reap its benefits. However, for those with kidney stones and urinary calculi, avoid consuming too much ragi as it could increase the oxalic acid levels in the body.

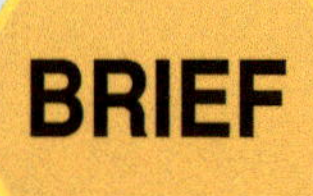

Preparation time: **20 Min**
Cooking time: **20 Min**
No. of servings: **4-5 Pc**
Fridge Life: **1 Day**

RAJGIRA (AMARANTH) PARATHA

Like nachni, rajgira is also a gluten-free, so since there is no gluten rolling them out evenly may take a while to make the roti. Use hot water for better results. This roti can be consumed during fasting or even during regular days. Though not commonly consumed as a paratha, rajgira paratha is satiating and wholesome. Serve with chutney or yogurt*.

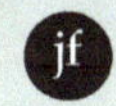 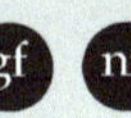 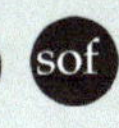 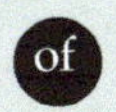 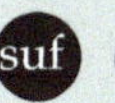 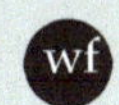

Ingredients

1. Rajgira *(Amaranth)* Flour (¾ Cup)
2. Jeera Powder or Whole *(Cumin)* (½ Tsp.)
3. Ginger-Chili Paste (1 Tsp. / Optional)
4. Freshly Chopped Coriander Leaves (3 Tbsp)
5. Hot Water to Knead the Dough
6. Boiled Potato (1-2 Pc Mashed/ Optional-Raw Banana)
7. Ajwain (1Tsp) (Carom Seeds)
8. Hing (1 Tsp)
9. Rock Salt to Taste

Tip: You can add dairy-free curds to further smoothen dough while rolling.*

** For dairy-free yogurt recipes, refer to **'Dairy Alternatives'** by Dr Rupa Shah, available on amazon.in and healthrevolution.in*

Method

- Put rajgira flour in a large bowl and pour hot water at the center.
- With a spatula, mix water gently in the flour.
- Let it cool a bit and add rest of the spices and mashed potato. Now knead the dough.
- Make balls from the dough. Roll-out parathas one a time.
- On a tawa, dry roast the parathas on both the sides just like roti. Do not use oil here.
- Serve hot with chutney or raita or potato bhaji.
- Optionally, add 1 or 2 boiled and mashed potato to the flour to make the parathas softer and flour stickier to hold together.

BRIEF

Preparation Time: **20 Min**
Cooking Time: **20 Min**
No. Of Servings: **4 to 5 Parathas**
Fridge Life: **1 Day**

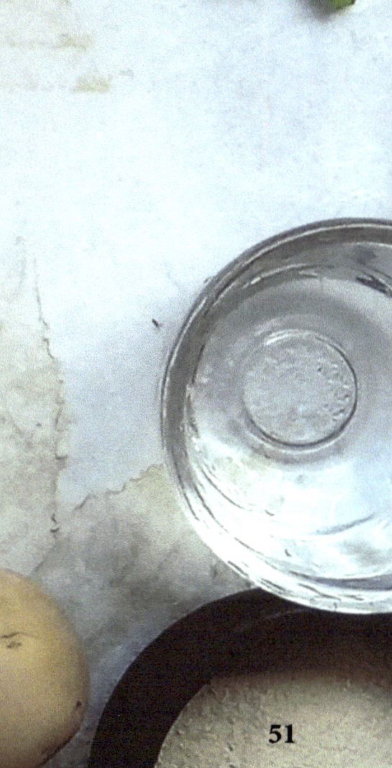

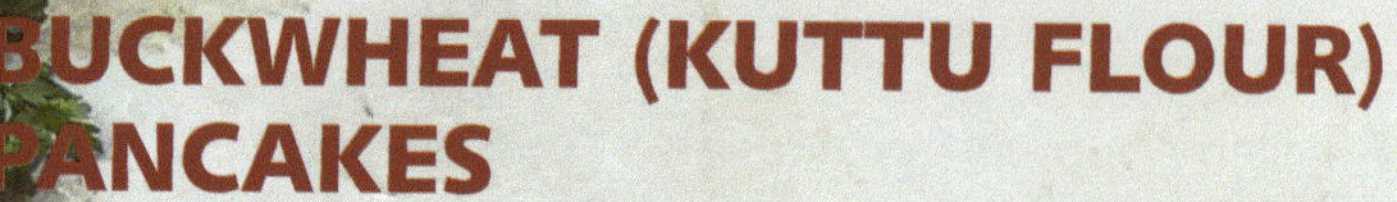

BUCKWHEAT (KUTTU FLOUR) PANCAKES

Pancakes are popular across the world. Try this Indian version of *kuttu* or buckwheat pancake, which is also called *chilla*. It is simple and easy to make. It makes a nice recipe for fasting days as well as a sustainable breakfast. Buckwheat pancakes are delicious and effortless.

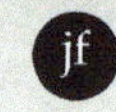

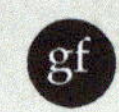

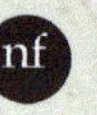

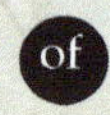

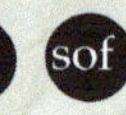

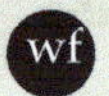

Ingredients

1. Kuttu *(Buck Wheat)* Flour (¾ Cup)
2. Fresh Water (1 Cup)
3. Green Chili (1 Pc/Finely Chopped) or Red Chili Powder (Optional)
4. Grated Ginger (1 Tsp /Optional)
5. Fresh Coriander Leaves (Finely Chopped /3 Tbsp)
6. Rock Salt to Taste

Method

- Mix all the ingredients well in a vessel–the batter should be 'dropping' consistency batter.
- Heat the dosa *tawa* (pan) well. Take a large spoonful of batter and pour it gently on the hot tawa. Do not spread it like a dosa (crepe), but more like a rawa dosa which is made by thinly dropping the batter on the tawa and let it spread on its own.
- Cook this pancake on medium heat. Once it is cooked on one side which may take 3-5 minutes, turn it and cook on the other side till light brown.
- Pancake is ready to serve. Eat hot.
- Serve with chutney, raita or bhaji.

Note: *Oil is not used while making this recipe.*

BRIEF

Preparation Time: **5 Min**
Cooking Time: **10 Min**
No. Of Servings: **3-4 Pancakes**
Fridge Life: **1 Day**

KER SANGRI (RAJASTHANI STYLE)

A local Rajashthani dish, Ker Sangri is a spicy *subzi* made with the ker berry and the sangri bean. Jains enjoy sangri and they consume it during Paryushan—a Jain festival involving a long fasting period. It is also a popular dish amongst Marwaris and Gujaratis across the world.

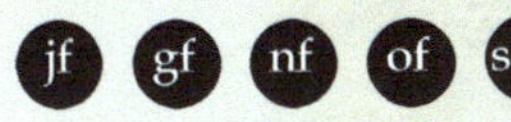

Ingredients

1. Ker (1 Or 2 Tbsp)
2. Sangri or Sangeri (1 Cup)
3. Jeera or Cumin Seeds (¼ Tsp)
4. Hing or *Asafoetida* (1/4 Tsp.)
5. Dry Kashmiri Red Chilies (2Pc/ Diced)
6. Turmeric Powder or Haldi (1/4 tsp.)
7. Red Chili Powder (1.5 Tsp)
8. Dhania Powder Or *Coriander powder* (2 Tsp)
9. Garam Masala (1 Tsp)
10. Amchur or *Dried Mango Powder* (1 Tsp)
11. Kismis, *Raisins* or (1 Tsp.)
12. Fresh Coriander Leaves For Garnishing (1 Tbsp/Chopped)
13. Rock Salt to Taste
14. Dry Dates (5 pc)
15. Jaggery (2Tsp)

Method

- Wash ker and sangri separately 4 to 5 times in fresh water. Now soak ker, sangri and dates separately overnight. Wash ker and sangri again in the morning.
- In a pressure cooker, combine ker, sangri and dates, with just enough water to steam for 2 whistles and then cook on low flame for 2 to 3 minutes. Let the pressure cooker cool off completely.
- Drain excess water and one more time, wash both in fresh water.
- In a pan, dry roast lightly the cumin seeds, asafoetida and red chilies for about 1 minute. Do not let it get burnt.
- Add the cooked ker-sangri, turmeric powder, chili powder, coriander powder, dried mango powder, jaggery, raisins and a little salt.
- Mix well and cook on a medium flame for 3 to 4 minutes, while stirring occasionally. Serve.

BRIEF

Preparation time: **10 Min**
Soaking time: **12 Hours**
Cooking time: **45 Min**
No. of servings: **1 Bowl**
Fridge Life: **4 Days**

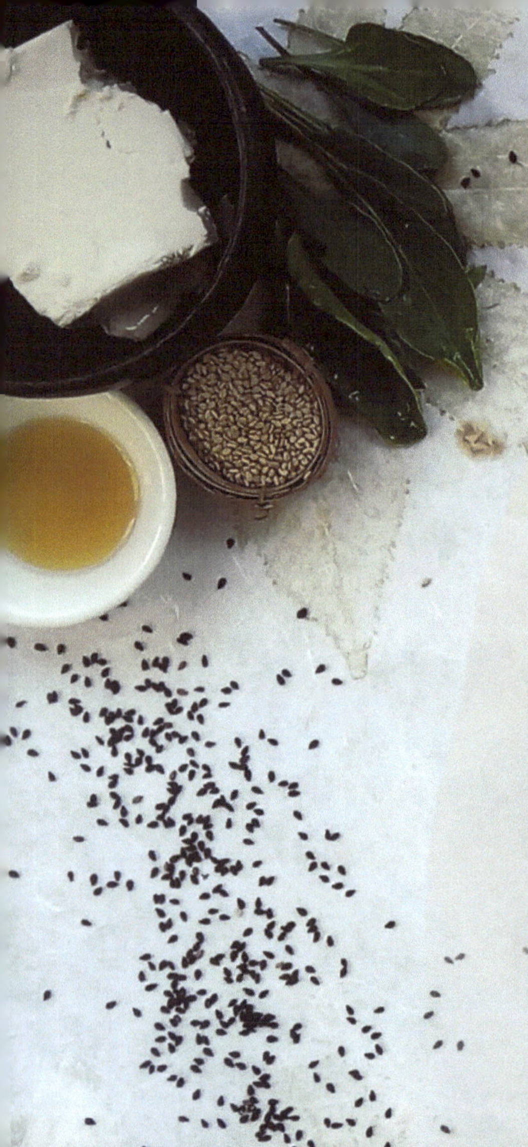

SPINACH, TOFU & SESAME STIR-FRY

Stir-frying is a popular Asian technique that can transform even the most insipid green veggies into tempting afternoon snacks. Try this spinach-tofu stir-fry that is loaded with calcium and will sooth the soul. The stir-fry is healthy and can be eaten with rice, quinoa or on its own.

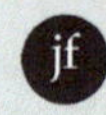

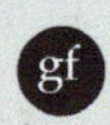

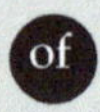

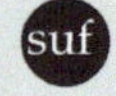

Ingredients

1. Tofu (Diced/ 2 Cups)
2. Baby Spinach or Spinach, Rinsed (Chopped)
3. White or Black Sesame Seeds (Roasted/ 2 Tbsp)
4. Garlic Clove, Minced (1 Large Pc)
5. Ginger (Grated or Minced /1 Tsp.)
6. Red Chili Flakes (¼ Tsp)
7. Soy Sauce to Taste
8. Rock Salt To taste

Method

- Heat a pan over low heat and add the diced-and-dried tofu.
- Stir-fry the tofu until it is lightly coloured, for 3-5 minutes, and add the garlic and ginger. Keep stirring for about a minute until they become fragrant.
- Stir in the soy sauce to taste.
- Add the spinach and stir-fry for a minute or until the spinach wilts.
- Add sesame seeds. Remove from the heat.
- Transfer the spinach and tofu mixture to a serving bowl, leaving the liquid behind in the pan.
- Add more soy sauce as desired.

Tip: You can serve with unpolished rice or noodles. It also makes a wonderful filling for whole wheat pita bread.

BRIEF

Preparation Time: **I.1Hrs.**
Cooking Time: **15 Min**
No. of servings: **4 Cups**
Fridge Life: **1 Day**

MULTI-SEEDS MUKHWAS

This recipe makes a handy post-lunch or dinner mouth refresher and a digestive aid. It is very rich in omega 3 fatty acids which are healthy fats and rich in calcium. The mukhwas helps build our cell membranes, signaling pathways and neurological systems. It is a calcium, magnesium & phosphorous-rich mix. If you have 1 Tbsp daily, it will contribute to overall health of bones, hair, and heart amongst other benefits.

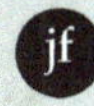

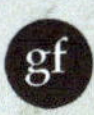

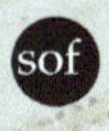

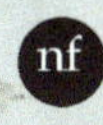

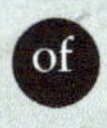

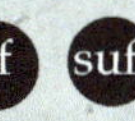

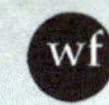

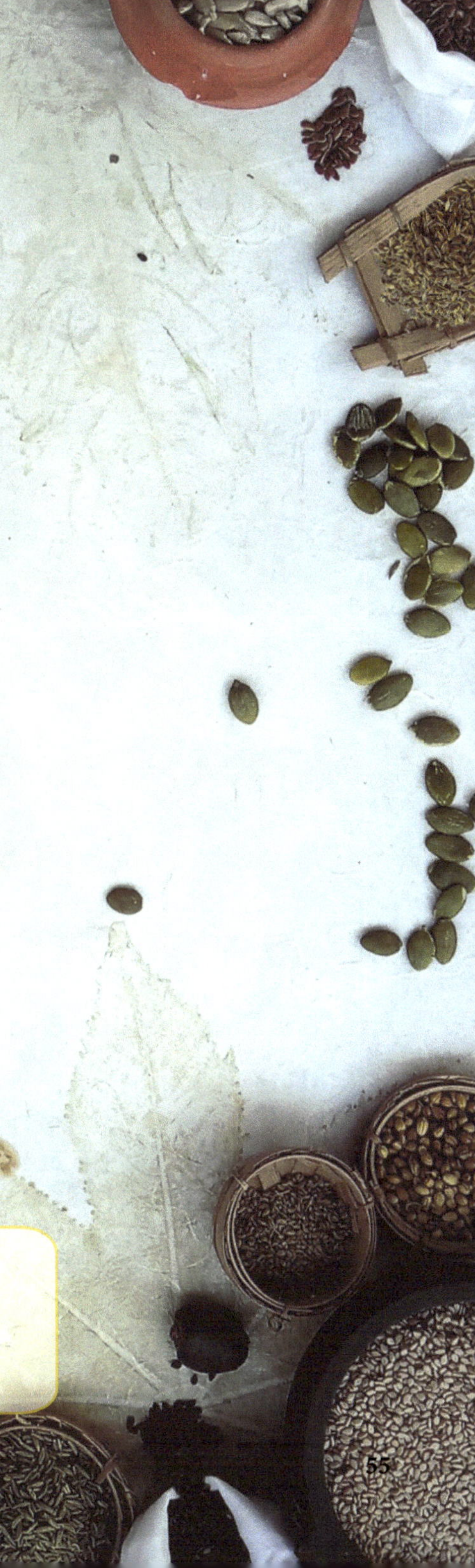

Ingredients

1. Flax Seeds (1 Tbsp)
2. Black Sesame Seeds (1 Tbsp)
3. White Sesame Seeds (1 Tbsp)
4. Fennel Seeds (1 Tbsp)
5. Coriander Seeds (1 Tbsp)
6. Dill Seeds (1 Tbsp)
7. Sunflower Seeds (1 Tbsp)
8. Pumpkin Seeds (1 Tbsp)
9. Ajwain or Thyme Seeds (1 Tbsp)
10. Rock Salt as Per Taste (½ Tsp)

Method

- Combine all the ingredients in a pan and lightly roast them.
- Cool and store in an airtight container.

Trivia: No meal is complete without the mukhwas. Many prefer it sweet, but try this earthy, nutty and crunchy recipe to re-boot your cells.

Note: All ingredients can be taken in flexible quantities as per personal preference.

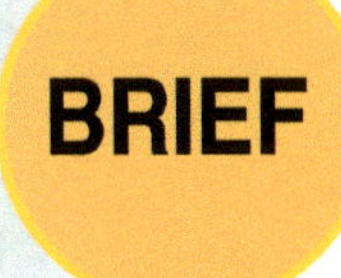

Preparation Time: **5 Min**
Cooking Time: **5 Min**
No. Of Servings: **100gm**
Fridge Life: **Not Required**
Note: Lasts for a month.

“Disease due to calcium deficiency is unknown in humans on natural diet.”

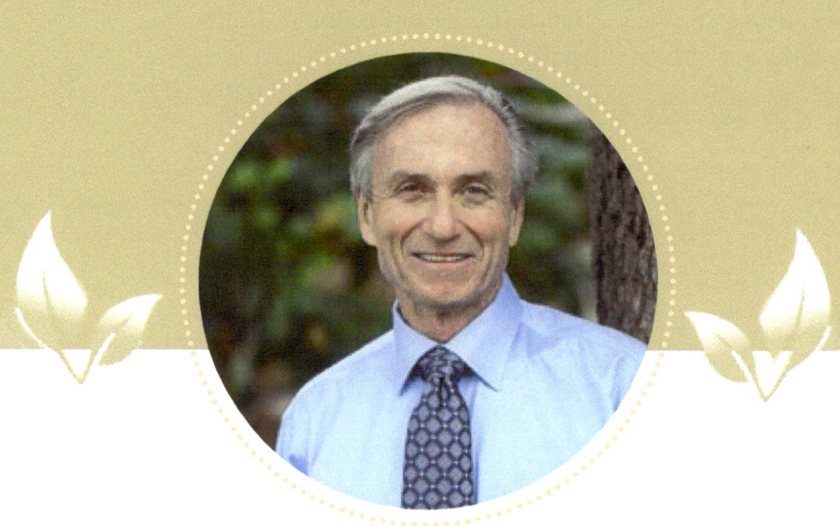

Dr John McDougall on Calcium

Much of what we have known about calcium or grown up believing may not be accurate. Dr John McDougall, a renowned expert on plant-based foods and author of several books has clarified many misconceptions about calcium in his books and articles. Here are the highlights

Are We Consuming Enough Calcium?

Many people worry that a diet without dairy products will lead to disease. The amount of calcium present in the diet has little effect on the quantity of calcium that is eventually absorbed into the body. “The intestine absorbs from the foods consumed sufficient calcium to meet the needs of the body. On low-calcium diets, the efficiency of absorption is increased, and on high-calcium diets less absorption occurs.”

Unprocessed vegetable foods contain sufficient calcium to meet the needs of adults and growing children. In fact, calcium deficiency caused by an insufficient amount of calcium in the diet is not known to occur in humans, even though many people in the world don’t drink milk after weaning because of custom, lactose intolerance, or unavailability.” Consider this the next time you hear the dairy industry’s favourite advertising pitch about the necessity of drinking milk to meet calcium needs.

Busting The Calcium Myth

The possibility of developing some vague illness imagined as "dietary calcium deficiency" haunts those not consuming milk and milk products. However, calcium deficiency of dietary origin is a myth and is virtually unknown in humans, even though many communities have walked this earth, have grown their normal-sized adult skeletons without the aid of milk (other than mother's milk during the first two years of life), and without concentrated calcium pill supplements.

Sources Of Calcium

The source of all calcium is the soils of the earth. All minerals, including calcium, come originally from the ground and enter animals through plants. This means plants are packed with calcium, iron, zinc, copper and so on, and the more plants you eat, the more minerals you acquire.

Animals do not eat the ground (or directly consume soil of earth), so how do they obtain this essential mineral? Plants absorb this basic element, present in watery solutions, through their roots, and then incorporate it into their various tissues—roots, stems, leaves, flowers, and fruits. Animals then eat the plant parts to obtain calcium and all other essential minerals.

Acting as the sole conduit, plants are loaded with minerals, in amounts sufficient to grow the skeletons of the largest animals that walk the earth, like the elephant, hippopotamus, giraffe, horse, and the cow. Since these massive bones can be formed from the raw materials of plants, you can assume there is sufficient calcium in vegetable foods to grow the relatively small bones of a human being.

The real reason we are losing calcium from our bones

In one long-term study, investigators measured calcium balance in adults and found that when subjects consumed as little as 75gm of protein a day, even with daily intakes as high as 1,400mg calcium, more calcium was lost in the urine than was absorbed into the body from the diet (a negative calcium balance). "This would mean that most westerners have a net loss of calcium from their bodies every day. The deficit must be made up from the body stores of calcium, which are primarily the bones. The end result of this continuous process is calcium-deficient bones that break with the slightest provocation, such as a sneeze that can crack a rib or a normal step that can break a hip. This condition is called osteoporosis, and in affluent societies it occurs in about 25 percent of women over the age of sixty-five. By the time of diagnosis, 50 to 75 percent of the original bone material has been lost from the skeleton."

Effects of Caffeine on Calcium

Excessive intake of caffeine may cause a rise in blood fats, a condition known as hypertriglyceridemia, which may contribute to illness. Cancer of the urinary bladder also has been related to caffeine use. One more undesirable effect of caffeine is that it has been shown to cause loss of calcium from the body. Therefore, a dietary maneuver you can use to prevent and possibly correct thin, calcium-deficient bones, or osteoporosis, would be to discontinue use of caffeine.

Protecting Your Bones

Sedentary people gradually lose minerals, especially calcium, from their bones. Inactivity eventually leads to a condition of thin, fragile bones or osteoporosis. This mineral loss is also affected by dietary factors and hormones. Exercise has actually been shown to increase the mineral content of bones.

References: 1) The McDougall Plan by Dr John McDougall 2) www.drmcdougall.com
Excerpts published with permission from
Dr John McDougall.

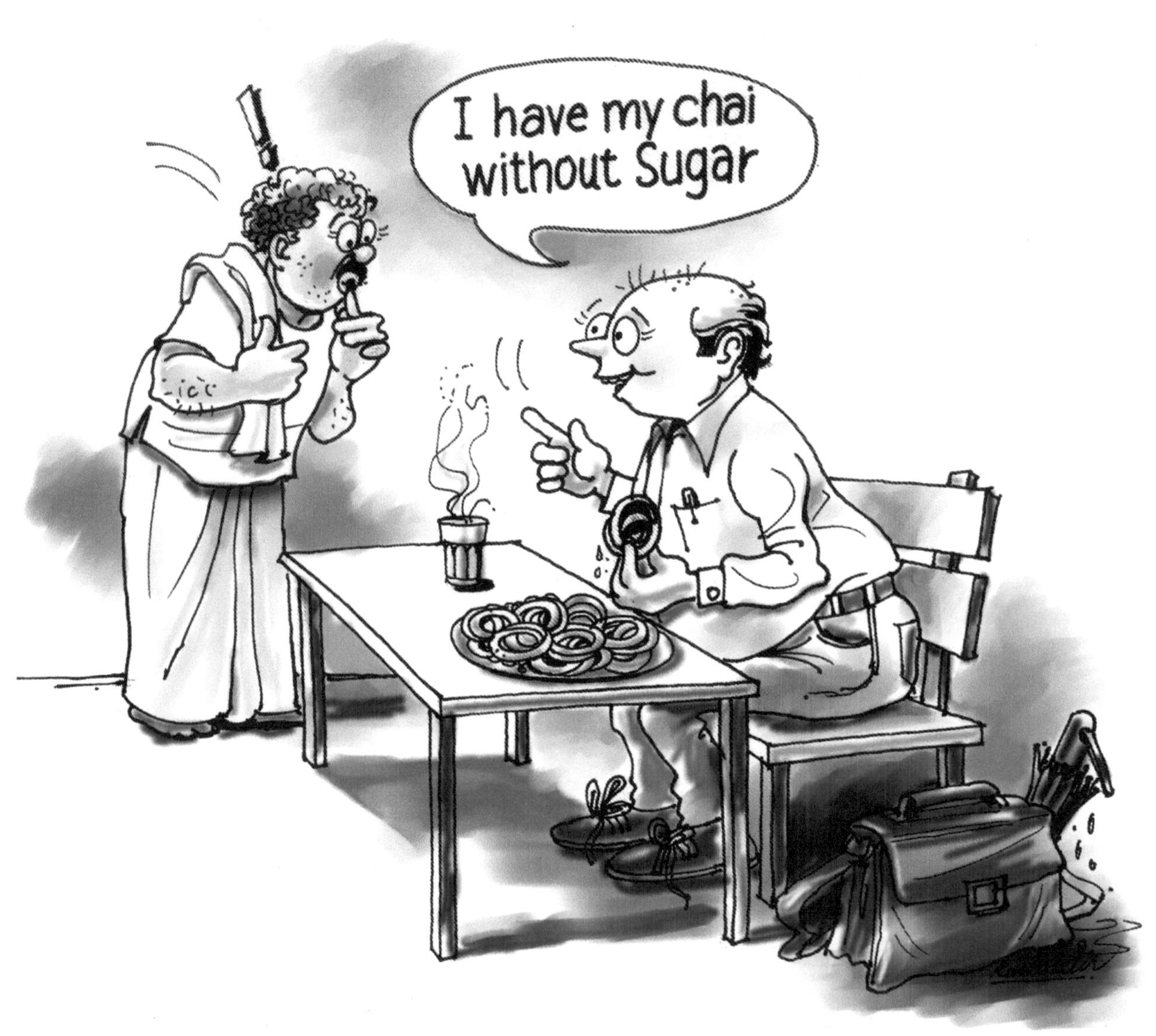
I have my chai without Sugar

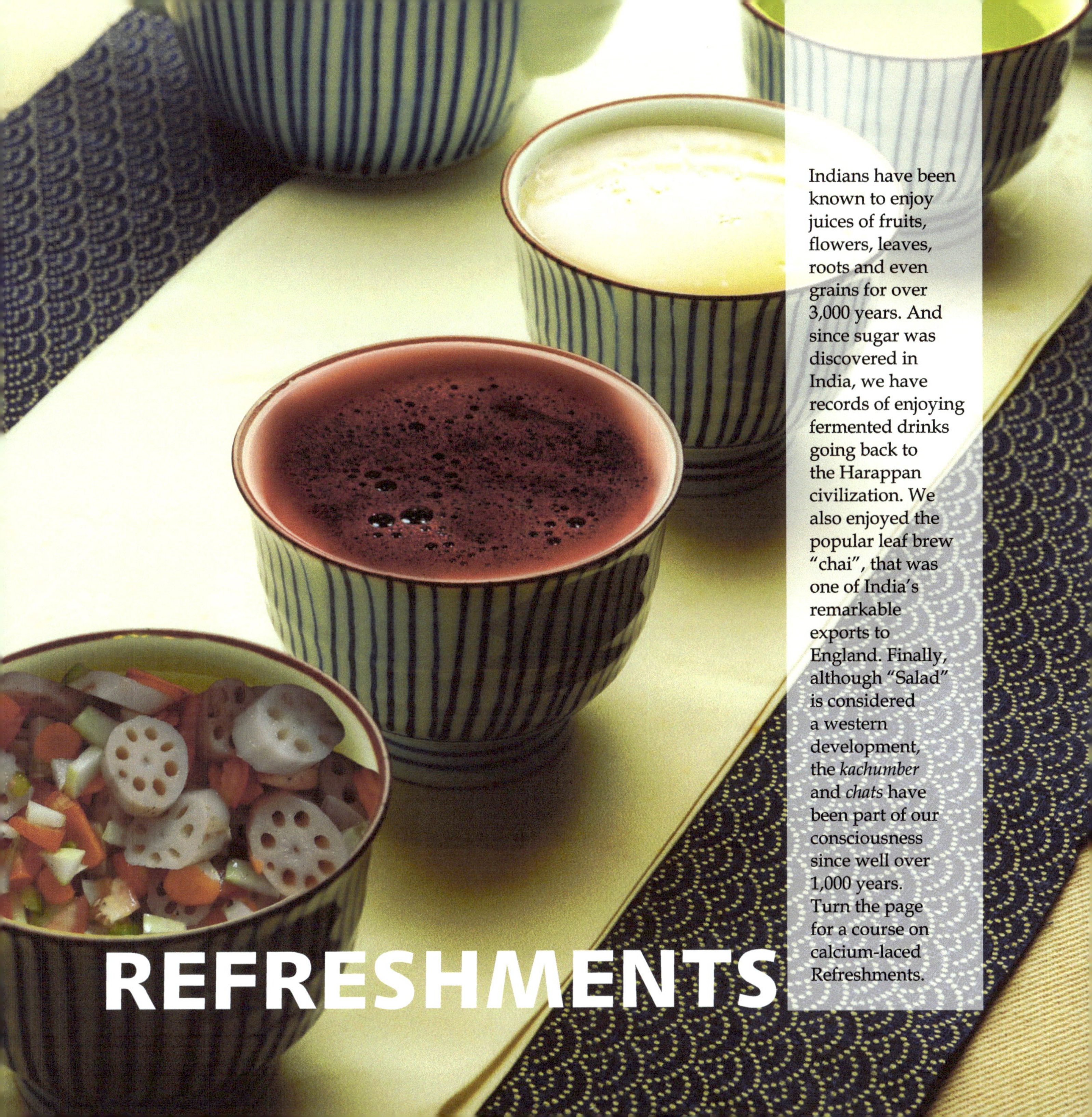

REFRESHMENTS

Indians have been known to enjoy juices of fruits, flowers, leaves, roots and even grains for over 3,000 years. And since sugar was discovered in India, we have records of enjoying fermented drinks going back to the Harappan civilization. We also enjoyed the popular leaf brew "chai", that was one of India's remarkable exports to England. Finally, although "Salad" is considered a western development, the *kachumber* and *chats* have been part of our consciousness since well over 1,000 years. Turn the page for a course on calcium-laced Refreshments.

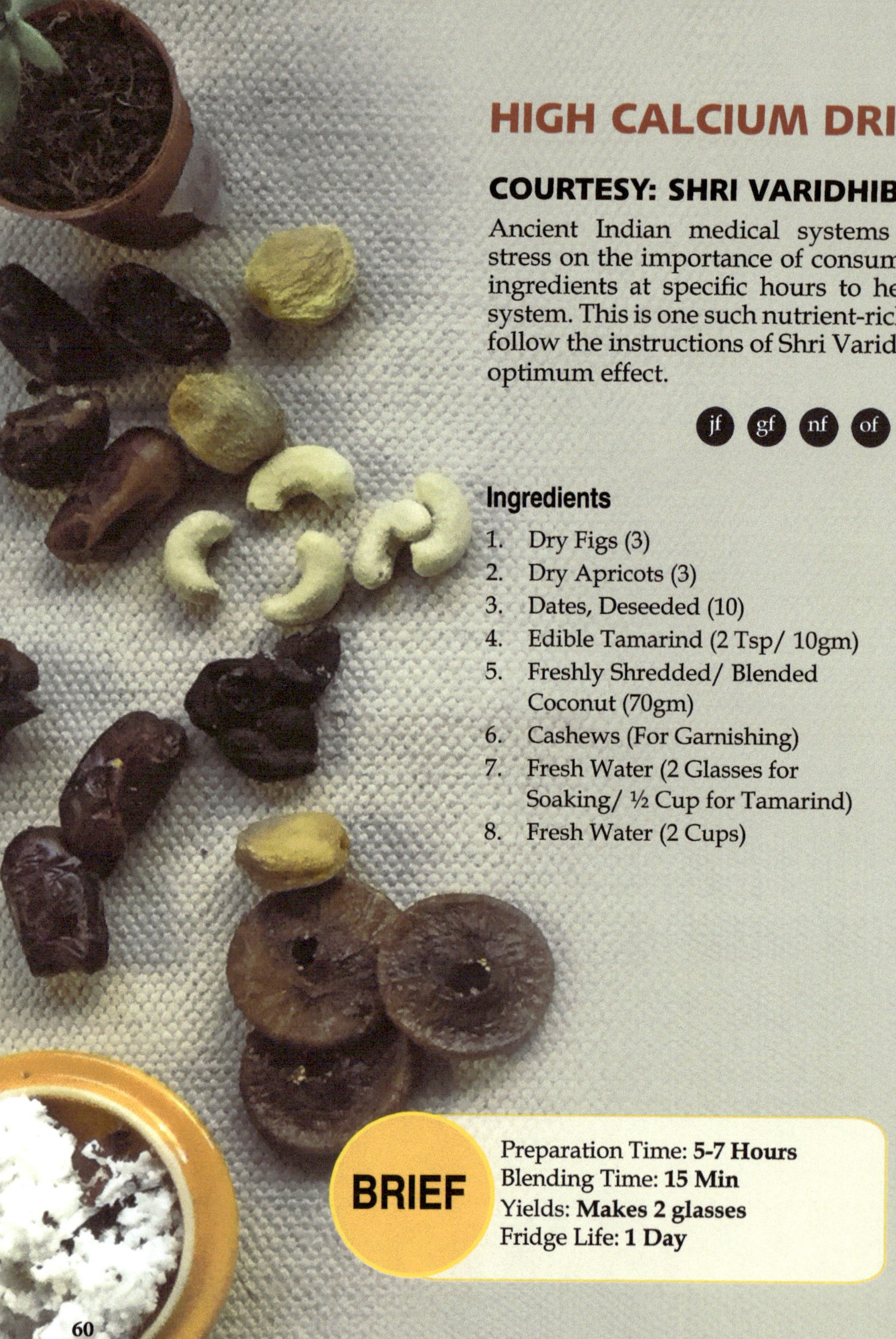

HIGH CALCIUM DRINK

COURTESY: SHRI VARIDHIBHAI THAKKAR

Ancient Indian medical systems like Naturopathy and Ayurveda stress on the importance of consuming specific drinks made of specific ingredients at specific hours to heal a malady or boost the immune system. This is one such nutrient-rich drink to boost energy levels. Please follow the instructions of Shri Varidhibhai, Naturopathy Doctor well for optimum effect.

jf gf nf of sof suf wf

Ingredients

1. Dry Figs (3)
2. Dry Apricots (3)
3. Dates, Deseeded (10)
4. Edible Tamarind (2 Tsp/ 10gm)
5. Freshly Shredded/ Blended Coconut (70gm)
6. Cashews (For Garnishing)
7. Fresh Water (2 Glasses for Soaking/ ½ Cup for Tamarind)
8. Fresh Water (2 Cups)

Method

- Wash figs, apricots and dates with clean water. Now soak these in 2 glasses of drinking water for 5-7 hours.
- Same way, wash tamarind and soak it in ½ cup water. Soak for 5 to 7 hours. Now squeeze tamarind in the same water and strain this water. Remove the fibre from the tamarind.
- Add this water to the water-soaked dry fruits.
- Add freshly shredded coconut. Blend the mixture in the blender.
- Drink is now ready. Garnish with cashews.

Tip: ***Replace tamarind with aamchur powder.***

Note: ***It is recommended to consume the drink 2 hours before meals or 5 hours after meals.***

BRIEF

Preparation Time: **5-7 Hours**
Blending Time: **15 Min**
Yields: **Makes 2 glasses**
Fridge Life: **1 Day**

LIME PEEL HERBAL TEA

Our local nimbu-paani *(sweetened lime juice)* is a household favourite beverage, especially during summers. But, how many of us know that if you throw in the lime peel, you get many alphabets like Vitamins C & A, and beta carotene, folate, calcium, magnesium and potassium as well! Lime peels contain as much as 5 to 10 times more vitamins than the lime juice itself. Chew on it!

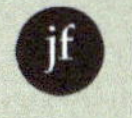

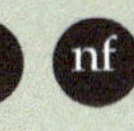

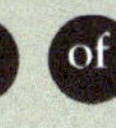

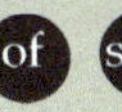

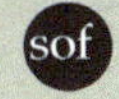

Ingredients

1. Peel of a Fresh, Organic Lime
2. Lime Juice (1 Tbsp)
3. Fresh mint (10 leaves)
4. Jaggery (1 Tbsp /Optional)
5. Fresh Water (600 ml)
6. Serves: 4 Cups

Method

- Wash lime well.
- Peel with a good peeler.
- Boil 600 ml of water in a vessel.
- In a kettle, first add lime rind at the bottom. Add jaggery.
- Pour hot water from the top.
- Let it rest for 10 minutes to cool.
- Add lime juice and fresh mint leaves.

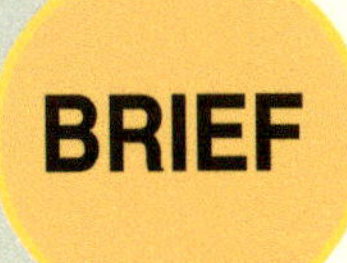

Preparation Time: **5 Min**
Blending Time: **15 Min**
Cooking Time: **Not Required**
No Of Servings: **2 Glasses**
Fridge Life: **1 Day**

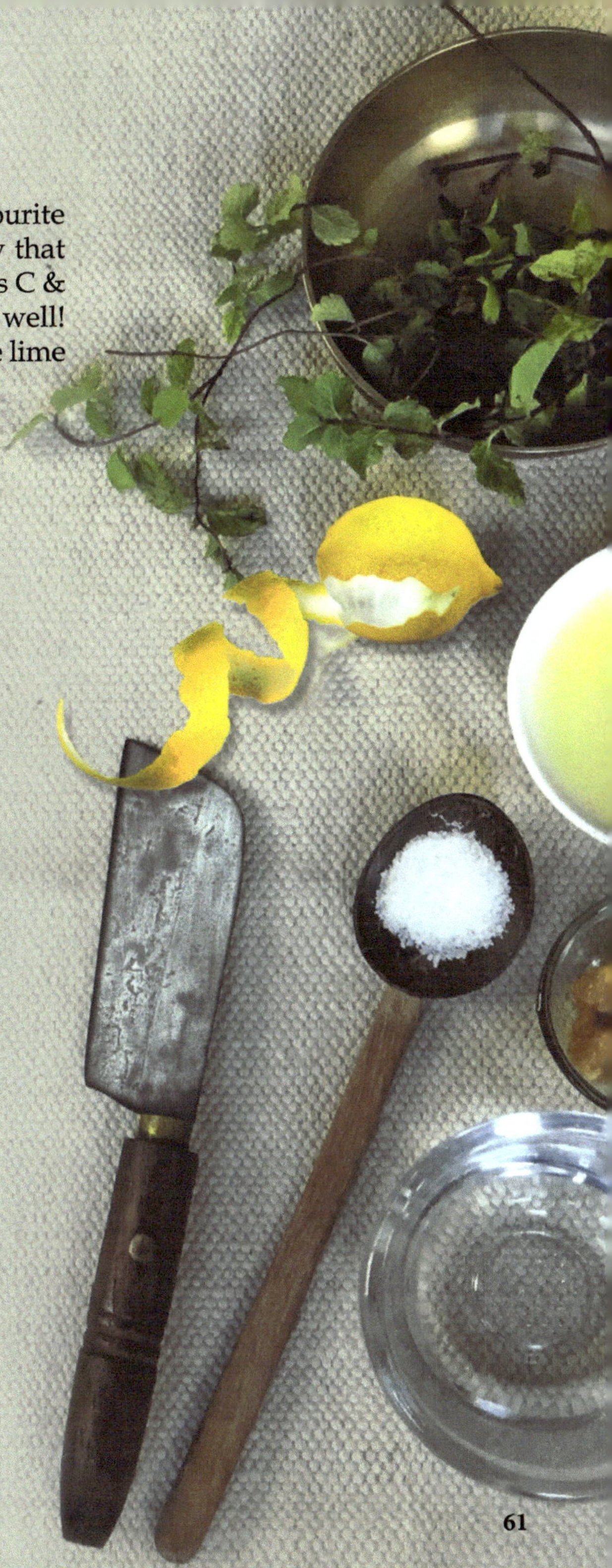

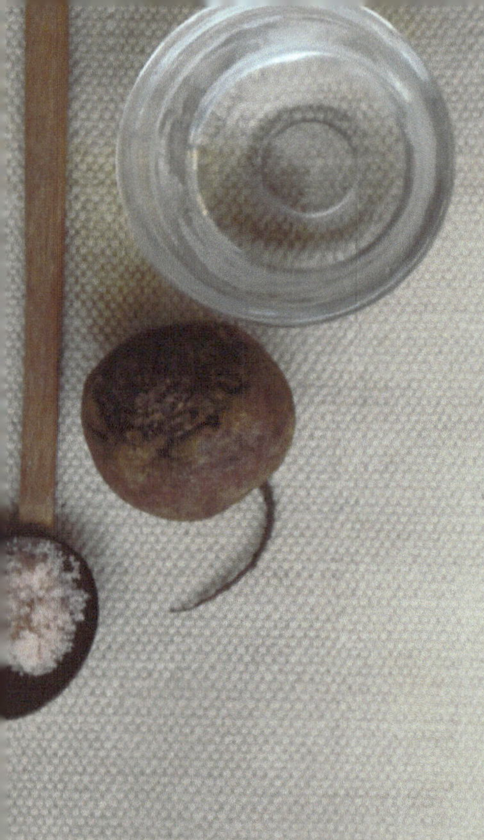

BEET 'GREENS' JUICE

Beet greens' juice is actually deep red in colour… and not green. The leaves of the beet plant are greenish outside but yield a red colour on blending. We often skip them as they have high levels of oxalates. Do not discard these leaves as they have a lot of other nutrients that are very good for you. Here we are using the leaves to extract juice.

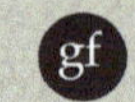

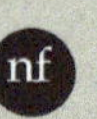

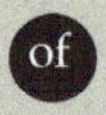

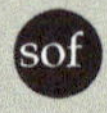

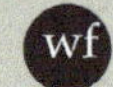

Ingredients

1. Beet Green Leaves (10 leaves)
2. Beet (1 Pc)
3. Drinking Water (2 Glasses)
4. Rock salt As Per Taste (Optional)

Method

- Wash beet and the leaves well.
- Cut the beet into small pieces.
- In a blender, add both. Blend well.
- Strain if desired.

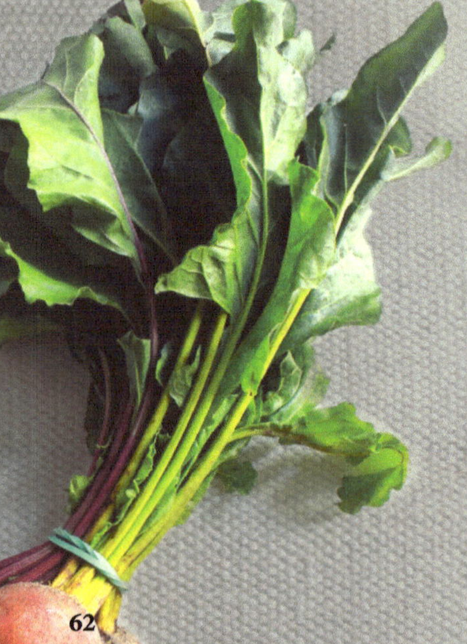

BRIEF

Preparation Time: **10 Min**
Cooking time: **Not Required**
No. Of Servings: **2 Glasses**
Fridge Life: **24 hours**
Note: Drink all juices fresh.

LOTUS STEM SALAD

Lotus stems are popular across South-east Asia, and are crunchy, fibrous and light. Also, owing to their neutral taste, they are incorporated into dishes ranging from salads and starters to main courses as well. This 13-ingredient recipe may be quite a handful, but keep going and you have a wholesome salad with a woody and fibrous taste that is rich with flavour and energy, and looks delicious.

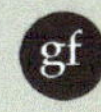

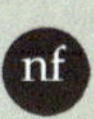

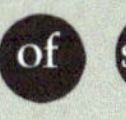

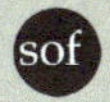

Ingredients

1. Kamal Kakdi (*Lotus Stems/ Bhein*) (1 Cup/ Sliced & Blanched)
2. Carrots (1 Cup/ Sliced & Blanched)
3. Cucumbers (½ Cup/ Sliced)
4. Red Tomatoes (½ Cup/ Chopped)
5. Celery (1 Tbsp/ Chopped)
6. Spring Onions for Garnishing (Optional)

For The Dressing

1. Lime Juice (2 Tsp)
2. Black Pepper Powder (Freshly Ground) To Taste
3. Raisins Or Date Syrup (3 Tbsp)
4. Soy Sauce (1 Tsp)
5. Rock Salt To Taste

For The Tempering

1. Cumin seeds Or Jeera (1 Tsp)
2. Curry Leaves or Kadi Patta (Few)

Method

- Blanch The Lotus Stem: Blanching is the process of removing the outer thin skin layer from the vegetable, without removal of the pulp. For blanching lotus stem, heat water to the first boil and cut the stem into three parts.
- Immerse the washed stem pieces to the boiling water for just less than a minute. Drain out the hot water.
- Remove the outer peel of the stem. Cut it into thin slices.
- For making the dressing, blend all the ingredients in a blender.
- Combine all the vegetables and dressing in a bowl and mix well.
- Dry roast the cumin seeds.
- When the seeds crackle, add the curry leaves and pour this tempering in the salad bowl and toss gently.
- Refrigerate for an hour and serve fresh.
- Garnish it with spring onions while serving.

***Tip:* Ensure that the inner surface of the stem is not torn. Blanched lotus stems can be used in sauteed salads.**

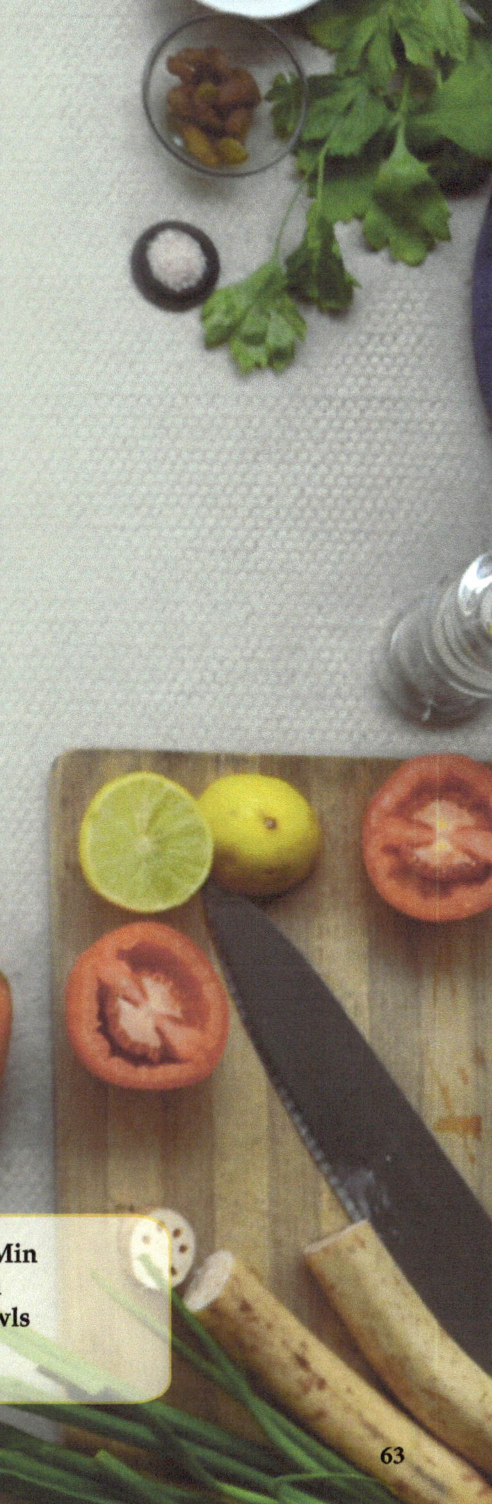

BRIEF

Preparation Time: **15 Min**
Cooking Time: **10 Min**
No. Of Servings: **3 Bowls**
Fridge Life: **4 Days**

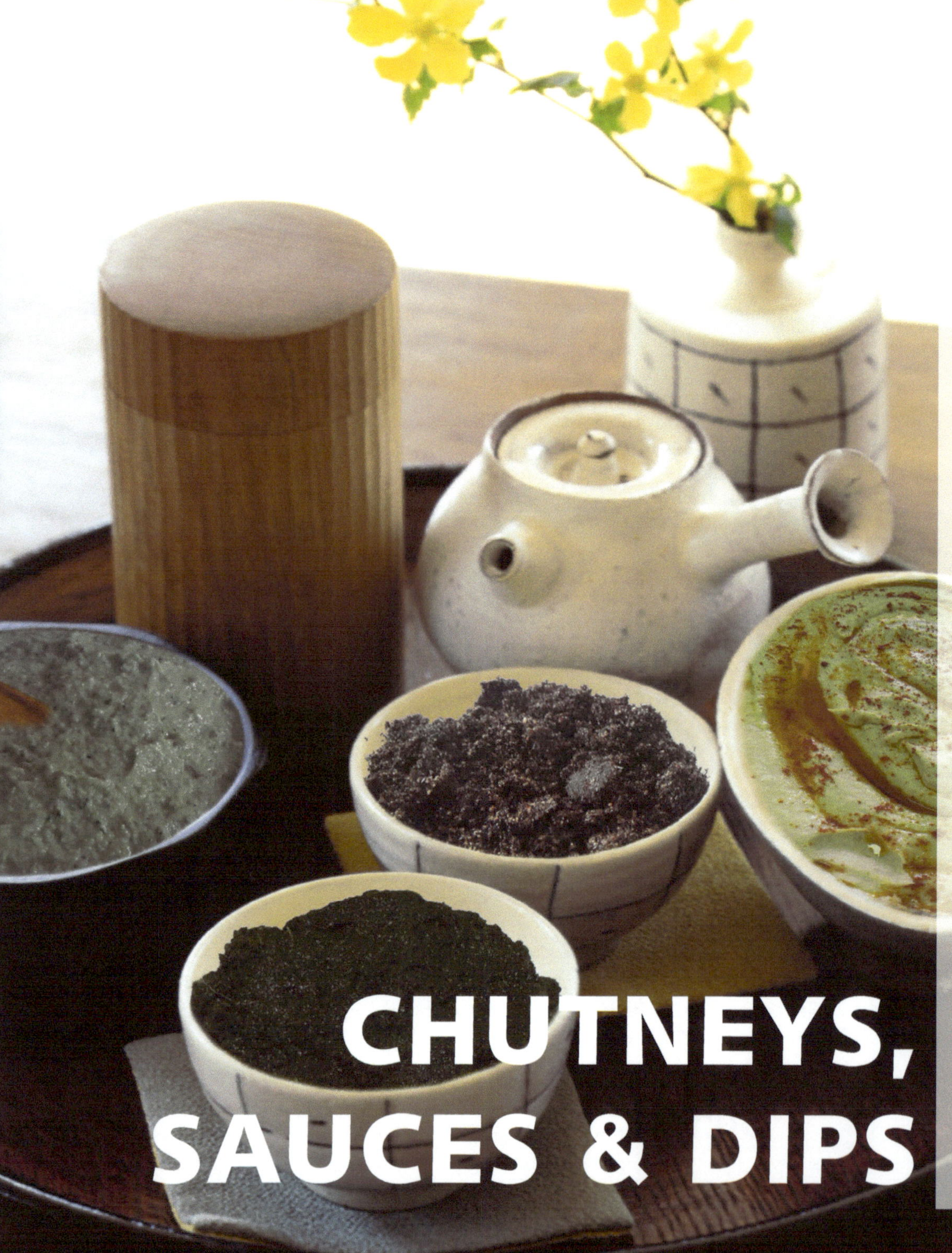

CHUTNEYS, SAUCES & DIPS

India has enjoyed condiments for over 3,000 years. Our civilizations have been known to use salt and lime for flavouring and preservation centuries before the word 'condiment' was even coined. Indians have made chutneys and have known the art of making fermented foods like pickles. It was only in the 17th century that chutney was exported to England and found its way into English dictionaries. Although there is no written record of our legacy of techniques that were surprisingly parallel to present-day physics and chemical engineering, many of our recipes have been handed down via generations. For this book, we have adapted popular sauces, chutneys, pickles and dips that are high on calcium and taste, while being easy to make.

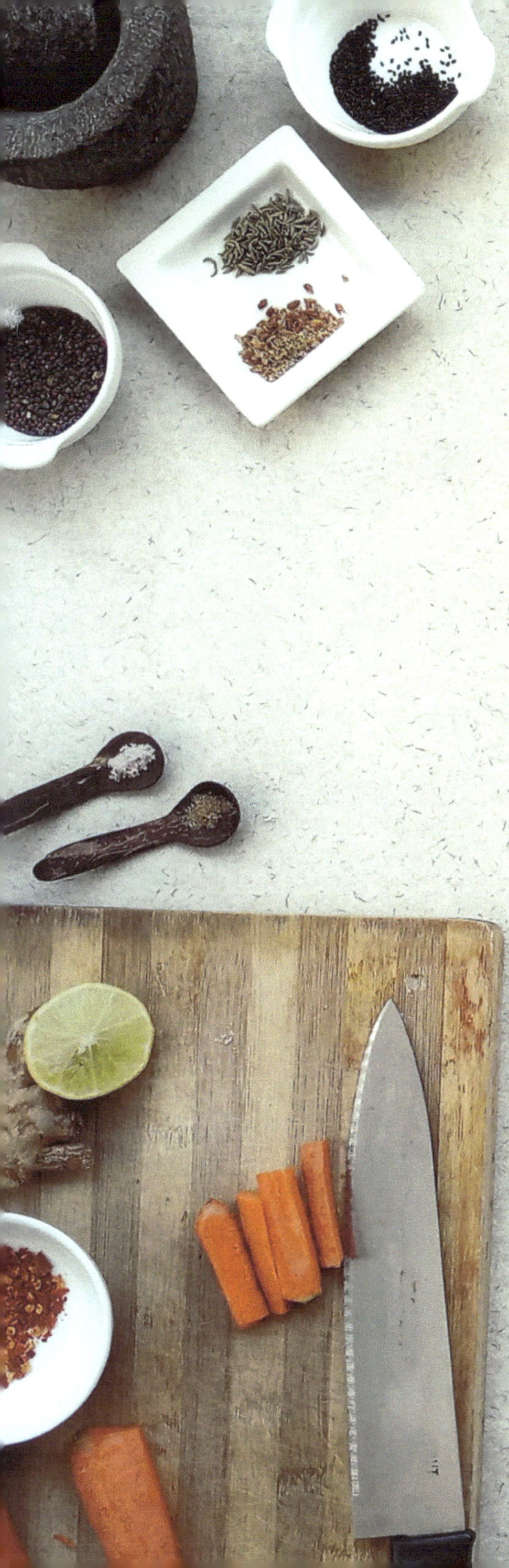

KALONJI & CARROT PICKLE

Black Onion seeds are also known as *kalonji* or nigella seeds. They are used in India and the Middle East as a seasoning for vegetables, legumes, salads and breads, samosa, kachori, namkeen and naan. Although the seed does not belong to onion family, it is rich in calcium. The black seeds taste like a combination of onions, black pepper and oregano, and have a bitterness to them like mustard seeds.

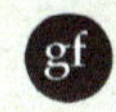

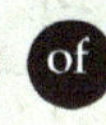

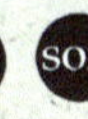

Ingredients

1. Carrots, Cut Into Julienne Or Small Finger Shapes (1 Cup)
2. Kalonji (*Black Onion*) Seeds, Coarsely Ground (½ Tsp)
3. Fennel Seeds, Coarsely Ground (½ Tsp)
4. Split Methi (Fenugreek) Seeds (2Tsps)
5. Split Mustard Seeds (2Tsps)
6. Hing (*Asafoetida*) (½ Tsp.)
7. Red Chili Powder (1 Tsp)
8. Turmeric Powder (¼ Tsp)
9. Ginger, Finely Chopped (Small)
10. Lime Juice (2 Tbsp)
11. Rock Salt to Taste

Method

- Mix all the ingredients in a bowl.
- Store in a glass jar and keep in fridge. Let it marinate for 1-2 days.
- Stir the pickle twice a day to prevent fungus formation

Tip: The quantities of the ingredients can vary as per personal preference.

BRIEF

Preparation Time: **15 Min**
Mixing Time: **2 Min**
No. Of Servings: **1 Cup**
Fridge Life: 1 Month

TAHINI DIP

Tahini is a condiment made from roasted ground hulled sesame seeds and is rich in calcium. It is widely used across Lebanese, Armenian, Greek, Israeli, Palestinian and Indian cuisines. It can be modified with lime juice, garlic, salt, red chili powder and other spices and used as dip or salad dressing.

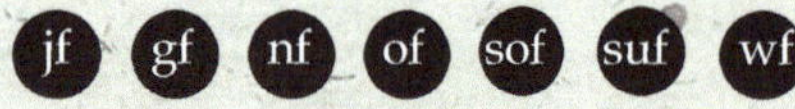

Ingredients

1. Lightly Roasted Sesame Seeds (1 Cup/ Can use unhulled or even sprouted sesame seeds)
2. Salt (Optional/ To Taste)
3. Black Pepper Powder (Optional)

Method

- In a small blender jar, add sesame seeds, about 1 inch in height. Blend it.
- Initially you will get powder of sesame. Continue to blend this powder for 1 or 2 minutes. Some amount of oil will release from this and the buttery tahini will be ready.

Note: Use hulled seeds for smoother texture.

Open Sesame!:

The sesame seed, the basis of tahini has been cultivated in Egypt since at least 2AD. However, tahini also appears in recipes from India, China, Vietnam and Greece that harks back to over 2,000 years. In most Middle Eastern cultures, the spread is called tahina, from the Arabic tahn, meaning "ground." but presently, Western countries use the Greek spelling, tahini.

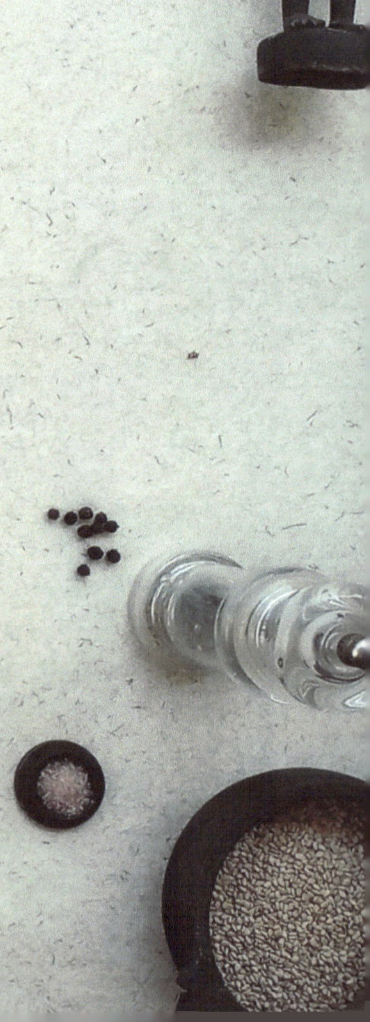

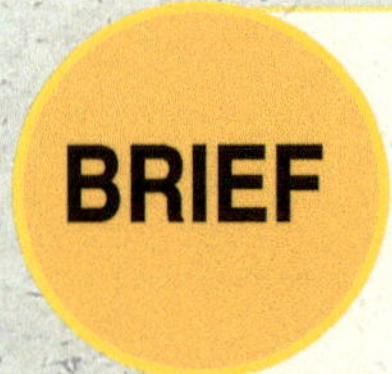

Preparation Time: **5 Min**
Blending Time: **5 Min**
Yield: **1/2 Cup**
No. Of Servings: **10**
Fridge Life: **1 Month**

WHITE BEANS HUMMUS (DRIED VAAL)

White beans, also known as white navy beans or *vaal* (in Hindi and Gujarati) and fava or lima beans, offer extraordinary health benefits. They are full of antioxidants, are low in saturated fat and sodium. It is also a good source of dietary fibre, protein, folate, iron, calcium magnesium, potassium and manganese.

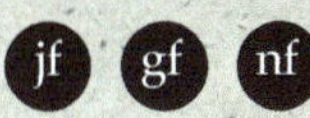

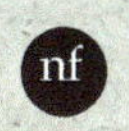

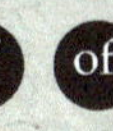

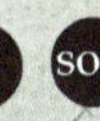

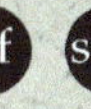

Ingredients

1. Dried Vaal or White Beans (1 Cup/ Soaked in warm water for 8 Hrs.)
2. Tahini (2Tbsp)
3. Lime Juice (1 Tbsp)
4. Garlic (1 Clove /Optional)
5. Onion Powder (1 Tsp/ Optional)
6. Red Chili Powder (For Garnishing)
7. Fresh Coriander Leaves (For Garnishing)
8. Water as per requirement
9. Rock Salt to Taste

Method

- Drain the soaked vaal and take fresh water.
- Boil vaal for 40 minutes until they are fully cooked. Can be pressure-cooked also. After they are ready, let them cool. Drain.
- Pour the cooked vaal in a blender. Blend well. Add all other ingredients except red chili powder and coriander leaves. Blend further.
- Add water if required to make it slightly thinner. It should be thicker consistency as such like a dip.
- Spoon out the dip in a nice glass bowl. Garnish with red chili powder and fresh coriander leaves.
- Serve with oil-free chips. Can be served warm or cold.

BRIEF

Preparation (Soaking) Time: **8 hours**
Cooking Time: **40 minutes**
Yields: **1 Cup**
No. Of Servings: **15 times**
Fridge Life: **1 Week**

SUNFLOWER SEEDS DIP

This makes a creamy dip that is perfect for crackers, chips, veggies, salad dressings and even as sandwich spreads. Also, it is one of our favourites, as it is easy to make and rich with calcium and Vitamin E.

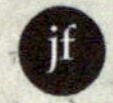

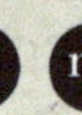

of
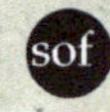

Ingredients

1. Sunflower Seeds (¼ Cup)
2. Water, 1-2 Tbsp & ¼ Cup
3. Lime Juice (½ Tsp)
4. Garlic, Peeled & Washed (1 Clove)
5. Dill Leaves, Cleaned and Washed (1 Tbsp)
6. Black Pepper Powder (Pinch)
7. Sea Salt or Rock Salt (¼ tsp)

Method

- Wash sunflower seeds well.
- Take a bowl and add sunflower seeds with ¼ cup water. Leave it covered for minimum of 8 hours and maximum of 10 hours. This will soften up the seeds. Drain.
- Add seeds to a blender jar with all other ingredients including 1-2 tbsp water. (More water will make it a thinner dip.) Blend well for about 2 minutes.
- Delicious sunflower seeds dip is ready to serve.
- Serve with cut veggies like carrots, cucumbers and radish.

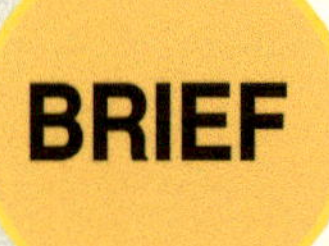

Preparation (Soaking) Time: **8-10 Hrs.**
Blending Time: **5 Min**
No. Of Servings: **1 Time**
Fridge Life: **7 days. Freshly made taste much better**

KARALE DRY CHUTNEY

Also known as *Kala Til* or *Ramtil, karale* or niger seeds are tasty and have many nutritional benefits. These seeds go by many names. In Kannada it's known as "*uchellu*" or "*gurellu*", and in Marathi it is known as "*khurasni*". Karale chutney serves as a good accompaniment with any meal and can be eaten with roti or rice. It belongs to the family of dry chutneys that are very popular in North Karnataka and Maharashtra. The chutney can be eaten anytime with healthy salads and snacks or with chapati.

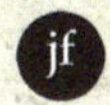

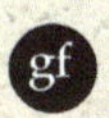

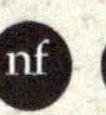

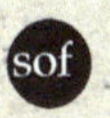

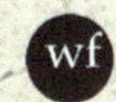

Ingredients

1. Karale (*Niger*) Seeds (100gm)
2. Garlic Pods (Peeled & Washed (6-7 Pc)/ Dry well With a Cloth.
3. Salt (1 Tsp. >) or As Per Taste
4. Red Chili Powder (1 Tsp/ As Per Your Taste)

Method

- Dry roast karale for 3 minutes on a slow flame stove in a wide-mouth vessel. Stir with flame on and off to make sure that they are well roasted and not getting burnt. Cut the flame and leave aside until cool.
- Dry roast garlic pods for 2 minutes in the same way. Remove from stove and let it cool.
- In a small chutney blender jar, add all ingredients and blend well.
- Dry chutney is ready. Store in an air-tight container.

Tip: **Freshly made tastes much better.**

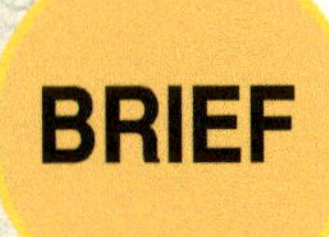

Preparation Time: **5 Min**
Blending Time: **5 Min**
No. Of Servings: **20 tsp**
Fridge Life: **30 days.**

CURRY LEAVES CHUTNEY

Curry leaves are available freely at your local vegetable vendor most of the times, yet its nutritional value is priceless. Don't take these common leaves for granted. They are more than just natural flavouring agents. The curry leaves have medicinal properties as they help in digestion, reduce acidity and indigestion, control diabetes and lower cholesterol. The chutney powder can be used anytime with salads and snacks like idli, dosa, khakhra or dhokla. Making dry chutney from these leaves is effortless. You just make it once and can relish it for many days.

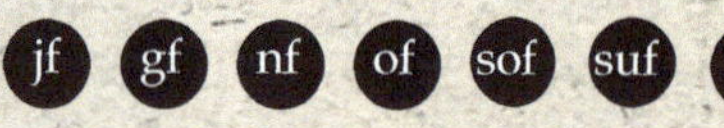

Ingredients

1. Dry Curry Leaves (Washed & Dried/ 1 Cup)
2. Garlic Pods, Peeled, Washed and Dried Well (6-7 pc/Optional)
3. Sesame Seeds (1 Tsp)
4. Red Chili Powder (1 Tsp.) Or As Per Taste
5. Black Pepper Powder (1 Tsp)
6. Coriander Seeds Powder (1 Tsp)
7. Aamchur (Dry Mango) Powder (1 Tsp)
8. Hing (Pinch)
9. Salt as Per Taste

Method

- Dry roast dry curry leaves 3 minutes on a slow flame in a wide-mouth vessel. Stir with flame on and off to make sure that they are well roasted and not getting burnt.
- Cut the flame and let it cool.

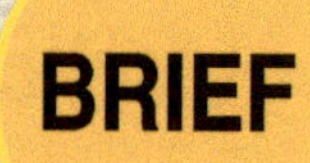

- Dry roast garlic pods for 2 minutes in similar fashion. Switch off the gas and cool.
- Dry roast sesame seeds for 2 minutes. Switch off the gas and cool.
- In a small chutney blender jar, add all ingredients and blend well.
- Dry chutney is ready.

Tip 1: Dry the leaves for well over an hour for best results.

Tip 2: Store in an air tight container for a longer shelf life.

Note: **Freshly made taste much better.**

BRIEF

Preparation Time: **5 Min**
Dry Roasting time: **6-7 Min**
Blending Time: **5 Min**
No. Of Servings: **10 times**
Fridge Life: **30 days.**

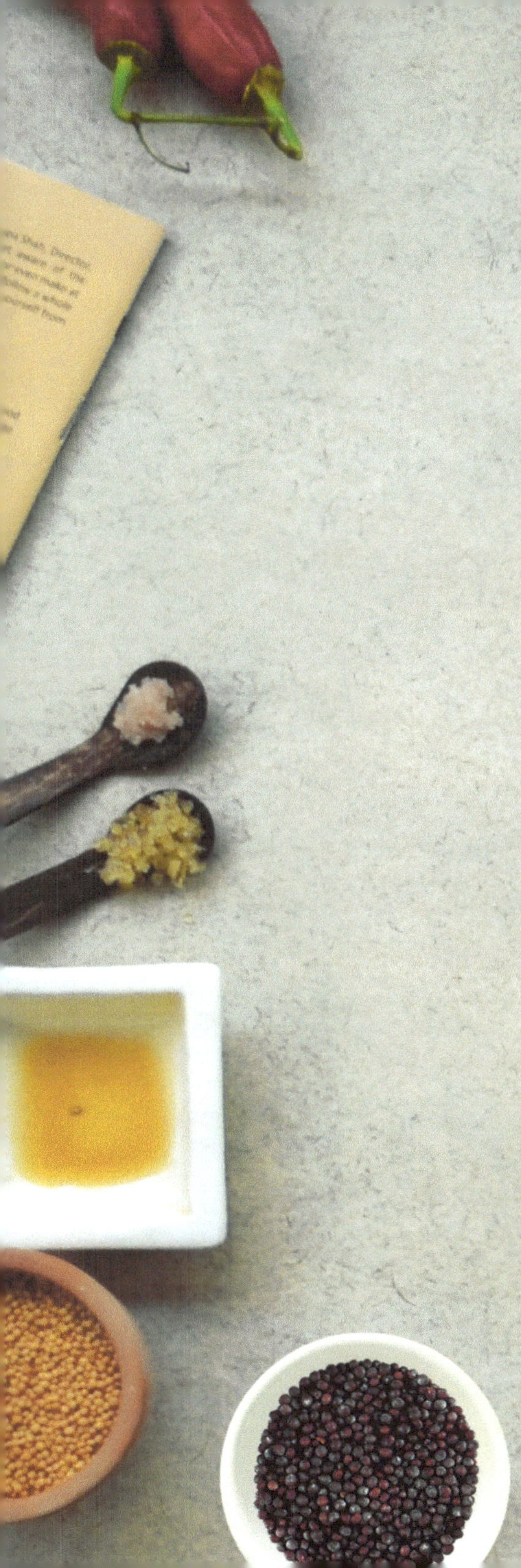

MUSTARD SAUCE

We either love it or hate it. Mustard (sauce is a thick yellowish-brown paste with a sharp taste. It is made from the grounded seeds of a mustard plant (black or brown/ yellow mustard seeds). Whatever you feel, you just can't deny that mustard is a tremendous powerhouse of nutrition. Although not part of this recipe, mustard greens or leaves are also excellent source of essential minerals including potassium, calcium and phosphorous, magnesium and dietary fibre. As a prepared sauce, it is still not compromised and is rich in nutritional value. Very easy to make, this healthy sauce can be used like salad dressing or spread or for sandwiches.

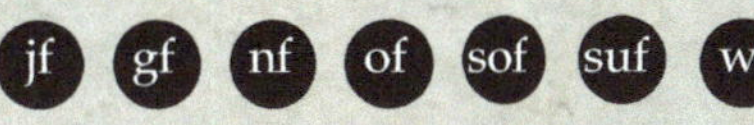

Ingredients

1. Sarson or Rai (*Black Mustard Seeds)* (250gm)
2. Yellow Mustard Seeds (125gm)
3. Whole Dry Kashmiri Red Chilies (5 to 6 Pc)
4. Garlic (4-5 Pods/ Optional)
5. Kakvi or Jaggery Syrup (1/2 Tbsp/ Optional)
6. Vinegar or Lime juice as required for grinding
7. Rock Salt to Taste

Method

- Except salt and jaggery syrup, blend all the ingredients well in a chutney blender.
- Add salt and jaggary syrup as per your taste.
- Add a little bit of more vinegar or lime juice to make it sauce like consistency.
- Store in a dry glass jar preferably.

Tip 1: You can also use lime juice instead of apple cider vinegar as mentioned before.

Tip 2: Use a dry spoon to serve the sauce.

BRIEF

Preparation Time: **5 Min**
Dry Roasting Time: **6-7 Min**
Blending Time: **5 Min**
No. Of Servings: **20-30 Tbsp**
Fridge Life: **30 Days**

BASIL PESTO SAUCE

Traditional pesto sauce is made of olive oil, pine nuts, fresh basil and garlic–spike that with non-dairy cheese* and is a healthy addition to any diet. While it is rather high in calories and fat, pesto offers a wealth of nutrients and a punch of flavor that many other sauces lack. When enjoyed in moderation, pesto can enhance your health and nutrient intake. You can replace pine nuts with watermelon seeds or even walnuts in the pesto.

jf gf nf of sof suf wf

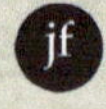

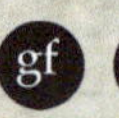

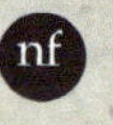

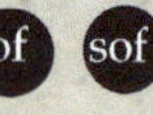

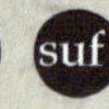

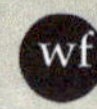

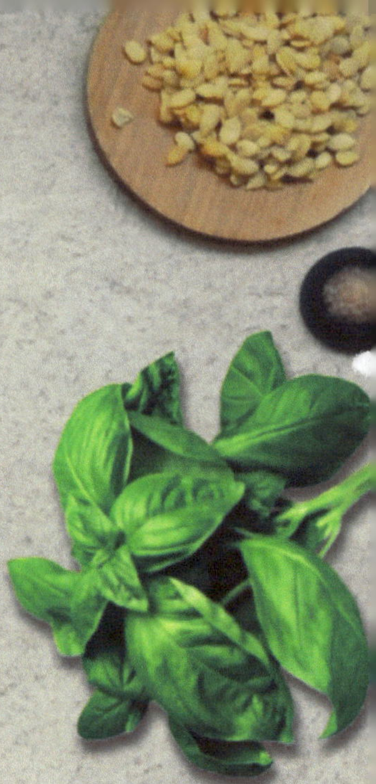

Ingredients

1. Watermelon Seeds (Magajtari/ ¼ Cup)
2. Garlic, Peeled (1 Clove/ Optional)
3. Basil Leaves, Washed (1 Tbsp)
4. Rock Salt (1 Tsp)

Method

- Blend all the ingredients for 3 minutes. Basil pesto is ready.

BRIEF

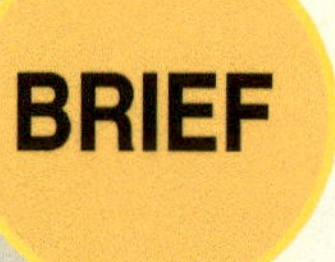

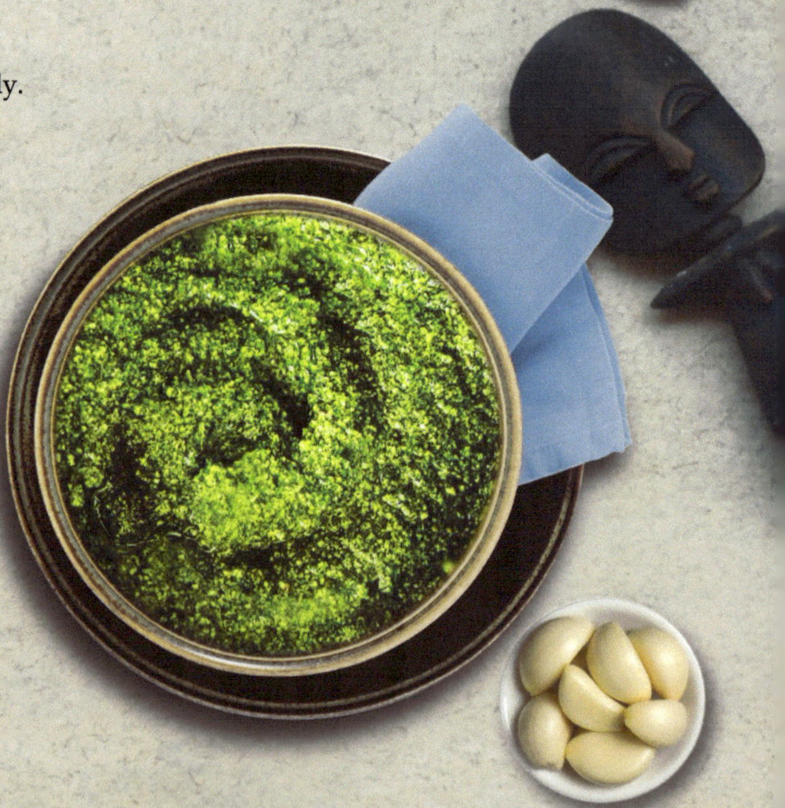

Preparation Time: **5 Min**
Blending Time: **5 Min**
No. Of Servings: **5 Times**
Fridge Life: **30 Days**

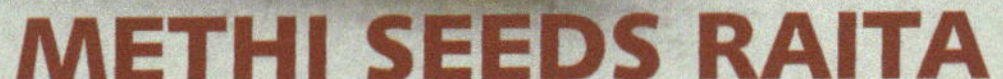

METHI SEEDS RAITA

Methi or *fenugreek* seeds have lots of health benefits which have been used as medicinal, therapeutic and natural home remedies for decades. They are widely uses in the kitchen for dals, parathas and curries. Methi seeds also make unusual, but tasty raita. It contains all the goodness of calcium of the methi seeds in an innovative way that is healthy and "finger-licking good "as well.

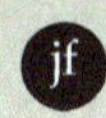

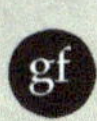

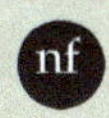

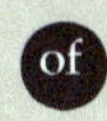

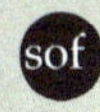

Ingredients

1. Dairy-Free Curd* (1/2 Cup)
2. Methi Seeds (*Fenugreek*) (4 Tbsps.)
3. Fresh Water (1/2 Cup)
4. Red Chili Powder (1 Tsp)
5. Natural Sweetener* (Optional)
6. Salt (1 Pinch/ Optional)

Method

- Soak methi seeds for 2 hours in ½ cup of fresh water. Throw away the water.
- Mix curd, methi seeds, salt and red chili powder. You can add a sweetener, but not necessary.

Tip: Serve chilled if possible.

* *Peanut-rice combo curd and soy curd offer best results.*

* *For natural sweetener recipes, refer to **'Dairy Alternatives'** by Dr Rupa Shah, available on amazon.in and healthrevolution.in.*

BRIEF

Soaking Time: **2 Hours**
Preparation Time: **5 Min**
No. Of Servings: **5 Times**
Fridge Life: **1 Day**

MAKHANA RAITA

Makhana raita is a nutritious and delicious accompaniment made from non-dairy curd and water-lily seeds. And if you love dairy-free curds* or yogurt, you just can't get enough of this dish. We were drooling while writing this recipe as well!

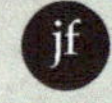

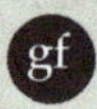

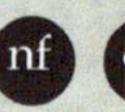

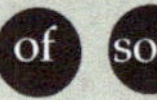

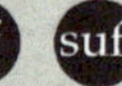

suf

Ingredients

1. Makhana (*Water Lily Nuts*) (1 Cup)
2. Non-Dairy Yoghurt* (1 Cup)
3. Roasted Cumin Powder (1 Tsp)
4. Black Pepper Ground or As Per Taste (½ Tsp)
5. Red Chili Powder (½ tsp)
6. Black Mustard Seeds (1 Tsp)
7. Coriander Leaves (1 Tbsp/ Freshly Chopped)
8. Black Sanchal (½ Tsp.) (Black salt) (Kala Namak)
9. Rock Salt to Taste

Method

- Lightly dry roast makhana in a flat pan for 2 minutes. Make sure you constantly stir the makhanas, otherwise it may burn too quickly.
- Lightly crush makhanas with hand blender or a regular blender.
- Add the crushed makhana into yogurt.
- Beat yogurt in a bowl.
- Add rock salt, black salt, cumin powder and black pepper powder and keep it ready.
- In a small pan, dry roast mustard seeds till it crackles. Turn off the stove.
- Add red chili powder.
- Add this seasoning from the pan to the raita and garnish with coriander leaves. Serve chilled.

* *For dairy-free curds or yogurt recipes, refer to '**Dairy Alternatives**' by Dr Rupa Shah, available on amazon. in and www.healthrevolution.in.*

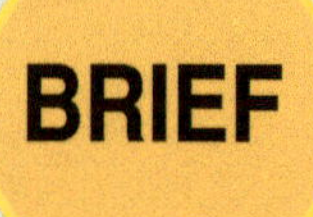

Preparation Time: **10 Min**
Cooking time: **2 Min**
No. of servings: **1 Bowl**
Fridge Life: **1 Day**

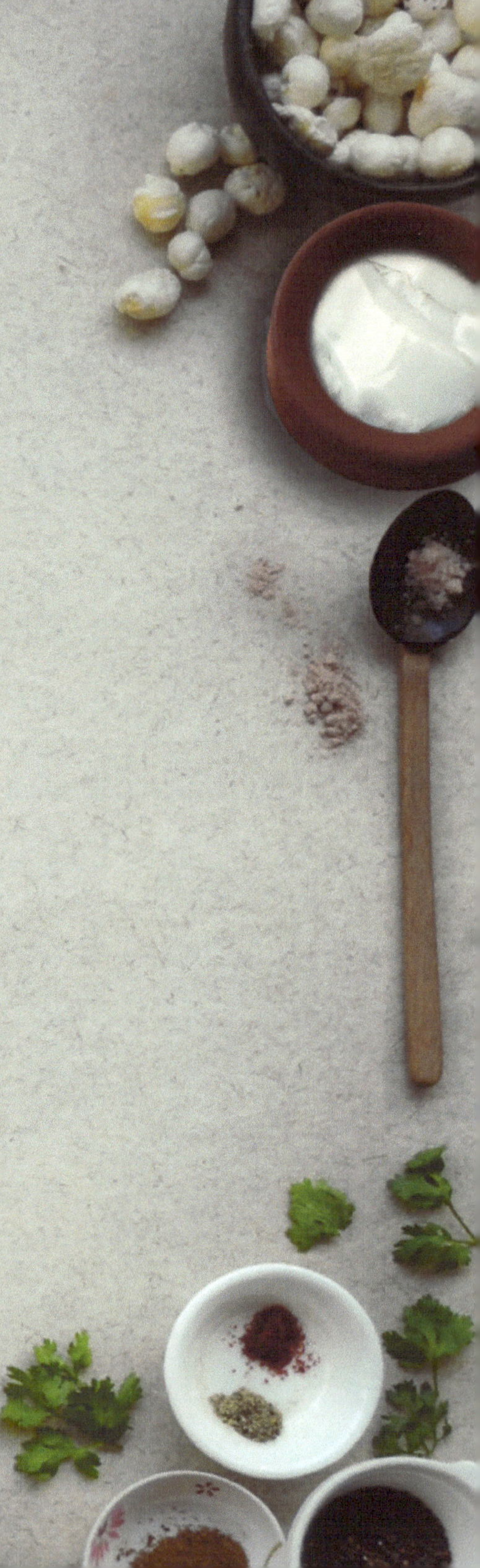

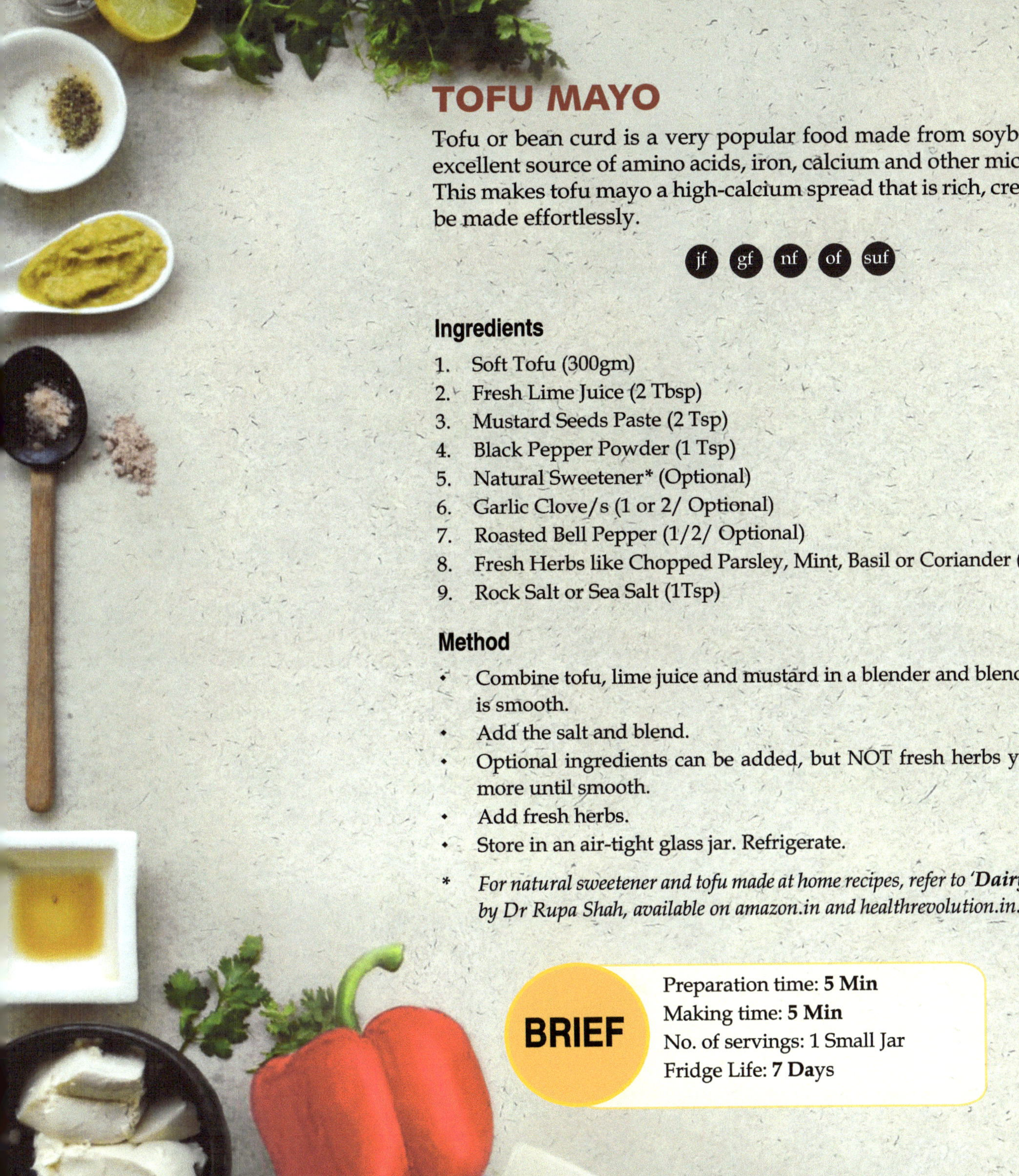

TOFU MAYO

Tofu or bean curd is a very popular food made from soybeans. It is an excellent source of amino acids, iron, calcium and other micro-nutrients. This makes tofu mayo a high-calcium spread that is rich, creamy and can be made effortlessly.

jf gf nf of suf

Ingredients

1. Soft Tofu (300gm)
2. Fresh Lime Juice (2 Tbsp)
3. Mustard Seeds Paste (2 Tsp)
4. Black Pepper Powder (1 Tsp)
5. Natural Sweetener* (Optional)
6. Garlic Clove/s (1 or 2/ Optional)
7. Roasted Bell Pepper (1/2/ Optional)
8. Fresh Herbs like Chopped Parsley, Mint, Basil or Coriander (Optional)
9. Rock Salt or Sea Salt (1Tsp)

Method

- Combine tofu, lime juice and mustard in a blender and blend until the tofu is smooth.
- Add the salt and blend.
- Optional ingredients can be added, but NOT fresh herbs yet. Blend once more until smooth.
- Add fresh herbs.
- Store in an air-tight glass jar. Refrigerate.

* *For natural sweetener and tofu made at home recipes, refer to '**Dairy Alternatives**' by Dr Rupa Shah, available on amazon.in and healthrevolution.in.*

BRIEF

Preparation time: **5 Min**
Making time: **5 Min**
No. of servings: 1 Small Jar
Fridge Life: **7 Days**

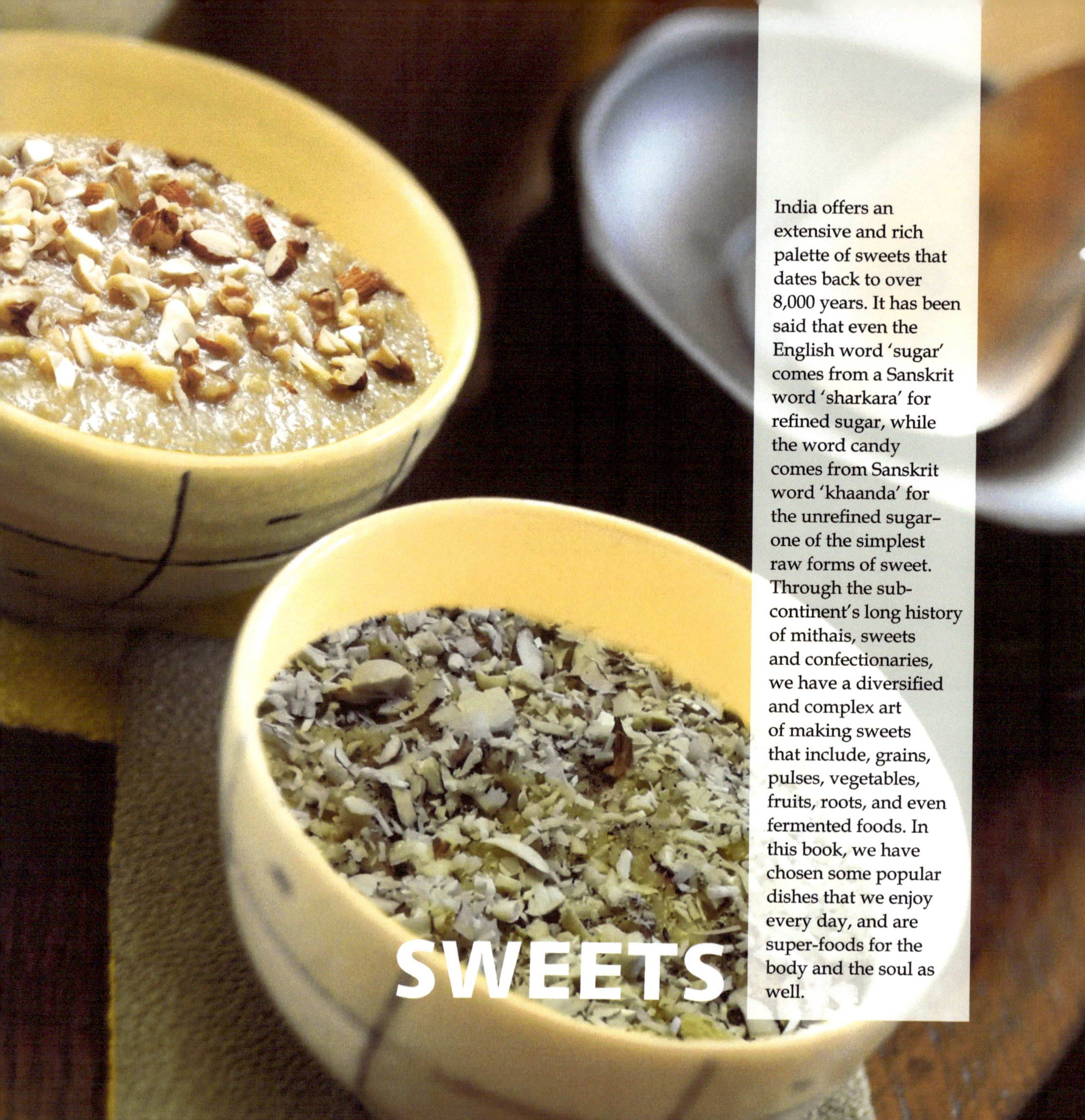

SWEETS

India offers an extensive and rich palette of sweets that dates back to over 8,000 years. It has been said that even the English word 'sugar' comes from a Sanskrit word 'sharkara' for refined sugar, while the word candy comes from Sanskrit word 'khaanda' for the unrefined sugar-one of the simplest raw forms of sweet. Through the sub-continent's long history of mithais, sweets and confectionaries, we have a diversified and complex art of making sweets that include, grains, pulses, vegetables, fruits, roots, and even fermented foods. In this book, we have chosen some popular dishes that we enjoy every day, and are super-foods for the body and the soul as well.

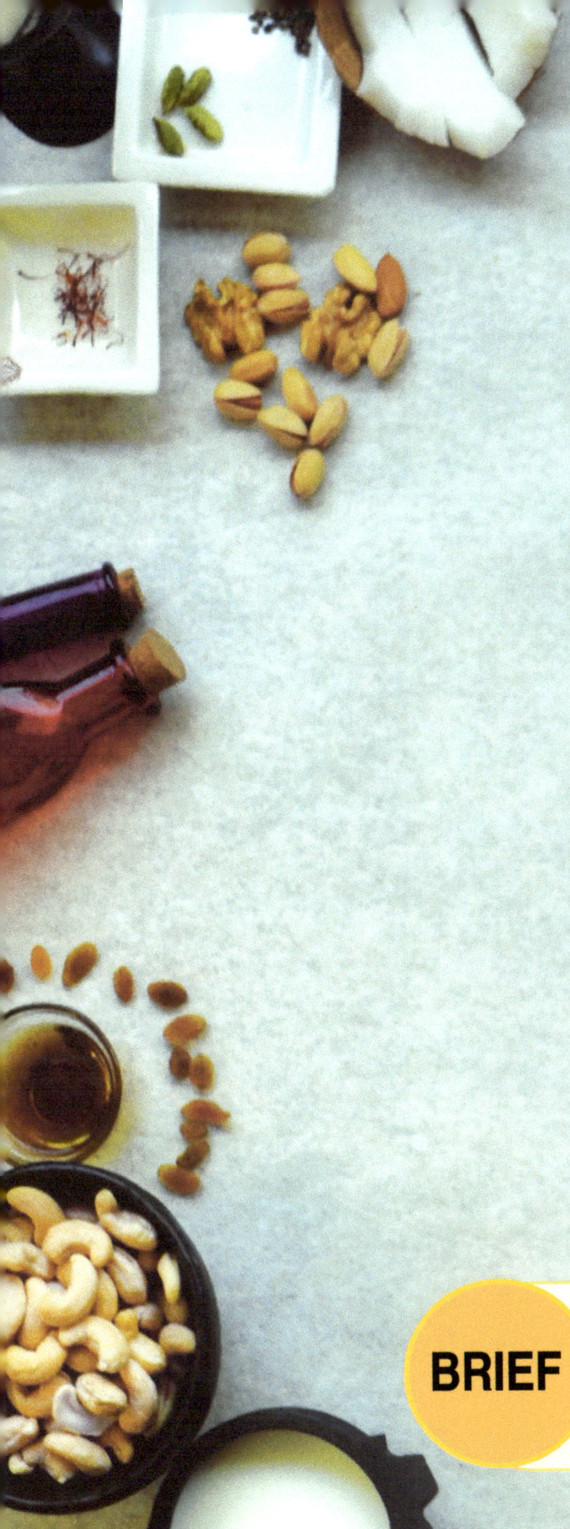

TOFU BARFI

Eating tofu as a sweet or a barfi may not be the first thing that strikes you, but this is a delicious and easy-to-make recipe. Offer this to your guests and you can expect expressions ranging from surprise to disbelief! Nevertheless, its effortless 20-min making time encourages people of all ages to try it more often. Not recommended for diabetics. Others, just beware that it can be addictive!

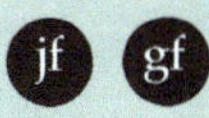

Ingredients

1) Unsalted Cashews (1 Cup)
2) Kakvi Syrup (½ Cup) or palm Sugar ½ cup
3) Shredded Fresh Coconut (2/3Cup)
4) Tofu (200gm/ Homemade Preferred)
5) Non-Dairy Milk* (< I Cup/ Soy, Almond or Any Other Milk)
6) Cardamom Powder (¼ Tsp)
7) Saffron (Few Strands/ Softened in a Tsp of water)
8) Chopped Nuts for Decoration

Method

- Make cashew powder in a dry blender jar.
- Crumble all the tofu in a dry blender jar.
- Mix all the 4 ingredients (cashew powder, palm sugar, coconut and tofu) in a broad pan. Cook on a slow flame for 5 minutes.
- Add dairy-free milk at this stage. Cook for another 5 minutes. The mixture will thicken.
- Add cardamom and saffron.
- After 1 minute, turn off the stove.
- Spread the mixture in a flat tray and let it cool.
- Add chopped nuts for garnishing.
- Cut into barfi shaped cubes and serve.

* *For dairy-free milk recipes, refer to* ***'Dairy Alternatives'*** *by Dr Rupa Shah, available on amazon.in and healthrevolution.in.*

Tip: **Freshly made tastes much better**

BRIEF

Preparation Time: **10 Min**
Blending time: **5 Min**
Cooking Time: **10 Min**
No Of Servings: **10 Times**
Fridge Life: **7 Days**

SESAME RAJGIRA & PEANUTS CHIKKI

An all-time favourite fast-food or snack-on-the-go, this mixed combination is very nutritious, healthy and a great way to kickstart or end your day. It may not be as light as popcorn, but you will love to bite this crunchy mix between meals or while watching your favourite flick or TV series.

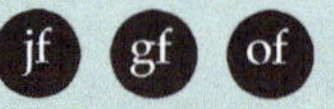
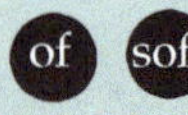
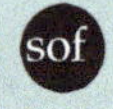
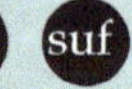

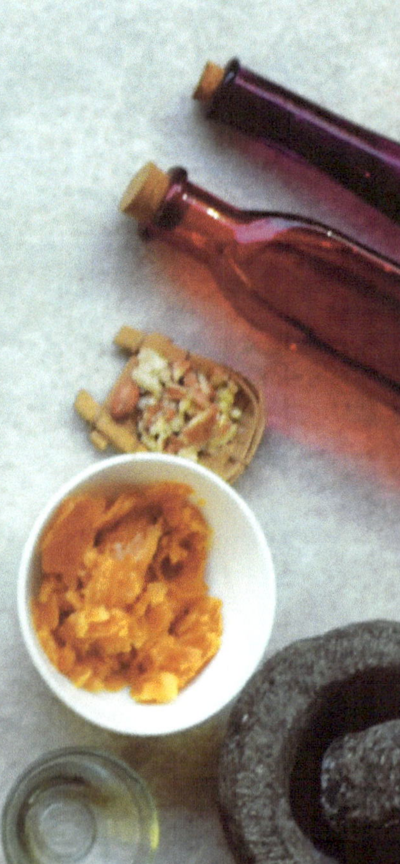

Ingredients

1. Rajgira (*Amaranth*)Puffs (3 Cups)
2. Roasted Peanuts, Semi-Crushed (2 Tbsps.)
3. Roasted White Sesame Seeds (2 Tbsps.)
4. Jaggery (1 Cup)
5. Fresh Water (1 Tbsp)

Method

- In a pan, take 1 tbsp water. Heat the pan for it a bit.
- Add jaggery and keep stirring for about 2 minutes until it melts and gets cooked (until you see it foaming). Turn off the stove.
- Add rajgira puffs, semi-crushed roasted peanuts and roasted sesame seeds.
- Spread this mixture on the steel flat dish and press evenly. With a knife, cut rows of chikki across the dish.
- Cool in for 3 hours outside.
- Store it in cool, dry, airtight container.

***Note:** Alternatively, with wet hands and bit of water, you can also roll laddoos out of the mixture.*

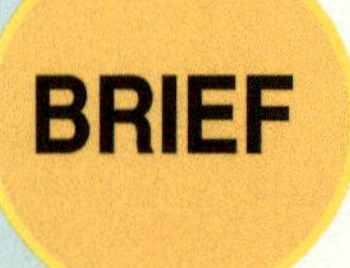

Preparation Time: **5 Min**
Cooking Time: **5 Min**
No. Of Servings: **15 Pieces Or 300gm**
Fridge Life: **Not Required**
Note: **Can keep outside for a month.**

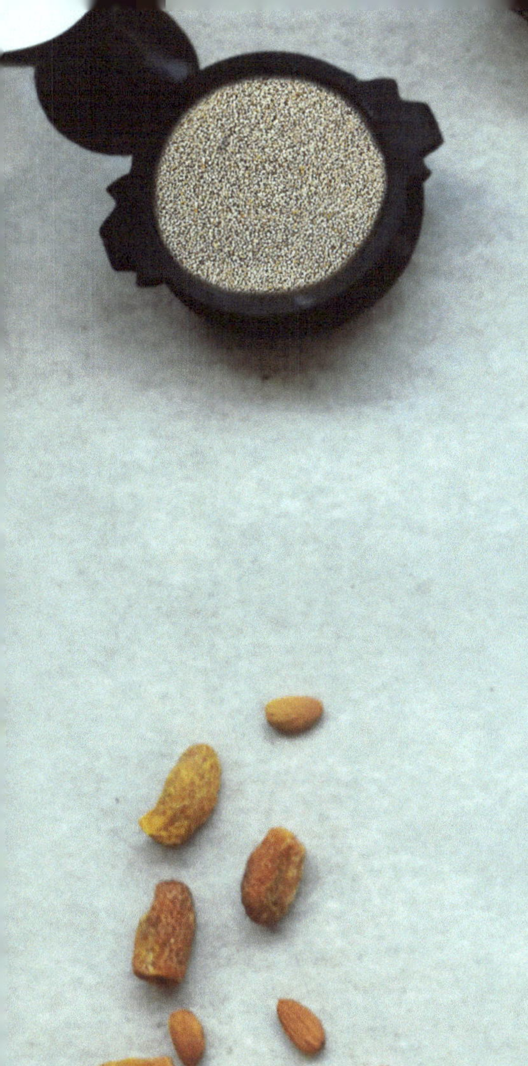

ALMONDS & POPPY SEEDS HALVA

COURTESY: JINAL RATHOD

Khuskhus (*poppy seeds*) halva with almonds is as irresistible to the tastebuds as to the eye. And its delicate, but rich aroma will leave you drooling. This halva is less gooey, and more textured like sheera. We have revised the recipe for this book. For first-time cooks, stay patient, you are sure to create a treat that is worth your while.

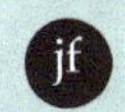

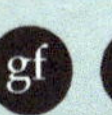

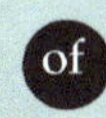

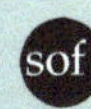

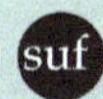

Ingredients

1. Coconut Milk* Extracted From Half Coconut (Brown Variety)
2. Khuskhus *(Poppy Seeds)* (1 Cup/ Soaked for 5-6 hours)
3. Kharek or *Dried Dates* (2 Cups) or As Per Taste (Finely Grated)
4. Cardamon Powder (6 Pods/ 1/2 Tsp. as Per Taste)
5. Almond Flakes for Garnishing

Method

- Rinse the khuskhus and blend till smooth.
- In a kadai, add the khuskhus paste. Start cooking. Stir constantly.
- Add coconut milk, little-by-little quantity and stir continuously.
- Add grated kharek as per taste in kadai.
- Cook until the coconut milk dries up and the halva thickens.
- Garnish with cardamom power and almond flakes. Serve hot.

Tip: Even chilled halva tastes good.

* *For dairy-free milk recipes, refer to* ***'Dairy Alternatives'*** *by Dr Rupa Shah, available on amazon.in and healthrevolution.in.*

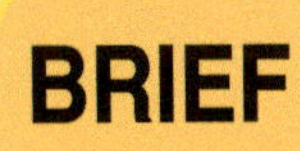

Preparation Time: **6 Hrs.**
Cooking Time: **20-30 Min**
No. Of Servings: **2 Cups**
Fridge Life: **15 days.**

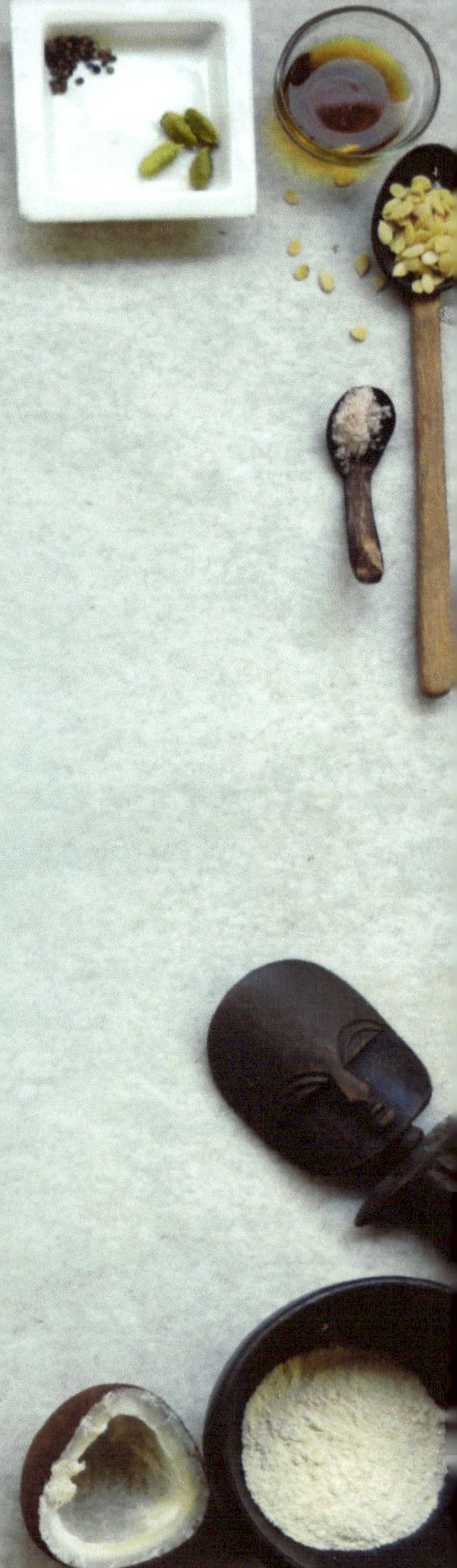

RAJGIRA GOLPAPDI

COURTESY: RICHA HINGLE

Rajgira is a quintessential fasting food made during winters, and it's loaded with fibre, calcium and vitamin C, and is easy to digest. This makes it a power food and if you make *rajgira golpapdi* (aka *sukhadi*), you now have a "power sweet". It makes a great post workout nutribar-cum-sweet and is easy to carry to work to bite into during those hours when you crave guilt-free sweets.

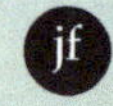

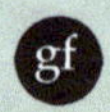

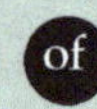

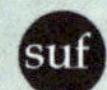

Ingredients

1. Rajgira *(Amaranth)* Flour (1 Cup/ *Rajgira* Atta)
2. Dry Shredded Coconut or Fresh Shredded Coconut (1 Cup)
3. Cardamom Powder (½ Tsp)
4. Kakvi Or Jaggery Syrup (12 Tbsp)
5. Watermelon Seeds for Garnishing (1 Tbsp.)
6. Rock Salt (Pinch)

Method

- Dry roast the rajgira flour in a pan for about 5 to 6 minutes on medium heat. Constantly stir the flour with a spatula until you smell the rich aroma of roasted rajgira flour.
- Add coconut flakes and mix well and cook a bit. Some amount of oil will separate from coconut.
- Add kakvi or jaggery syrup to this mixture. Mix fast and well. Don't cook for more than a minute. The mixture will be soft and spreadable consistency.
- Spread the mixture in a flat dish.
- Decorate with watermelon seeds. Let it cool.
- Cut into diamond pieces. It is ready to be served.

Note: It will be softer than regular golpapdi made with wheat flour.

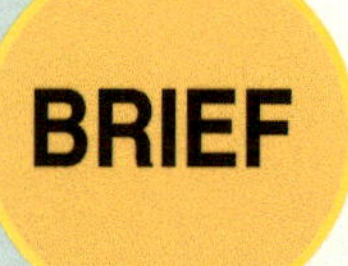

Preparation Time: **15 Min**
Cooking Time: **10 Min**
No. Of Servings: **30 Squares (Approx.)**
Fridge Life: **1 Week**

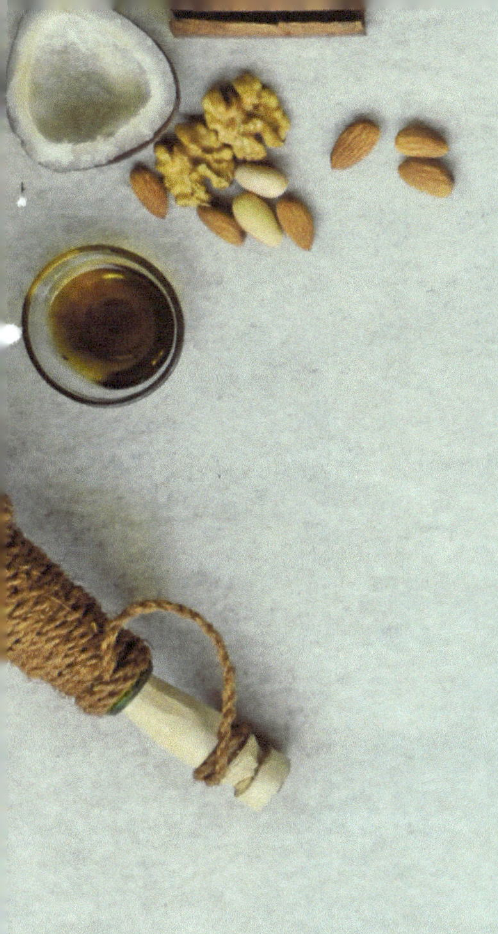

CHIA SEEDS PUDDING

Chia seeds are mini powerhouses, packed with calcium, Omega-3 and antioxidants. Because of their gel-like texture and ability to thicken they are a favourite when making desserts or milkshakes. It's very easy to make and has enough protein and nutrients to alternate as a quick, on-the-go breakfast option. This versatile dish that can be eaten for both breakfast and dessert, claims its top spot in the delicious, healthy snacks category.

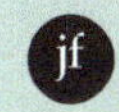

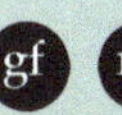

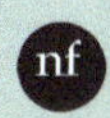

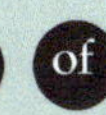

sof
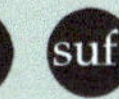

Ingredients

1. Unsweetened Almond Milk* Or Soy Milk (3 cups)
2. Chia Seeds (1/2 Cup)
3. Natural Sweetener like Date Paste or Raisins Paste (1-3 Tbsp. or to taste)

Suggested Toppings

Coconut Flakes
Cinnamon Powder As Per Taste
Nuts And Seeds
Banana Pieces
Cacao or Raw Chocolate Powder as Per Taste

Method

- Mix almond or soy milk, chia seeds and sweetener together in a large bowl. Let sit for 10 minutes and then mix again with a spatula. This helps prevent clumping.
- Cover and chill in the fridge for 4 to 5 hours, or overnight.
- Stir well and now add other toppings.
- Serve in glass bowls.
- Remaining pudding can be kept in an air-tight container in the fridge for 3 days.

* *For dairy-free milk recipes, refer to '**Dairy Alternatives**' by Dr Rupa Shah, available on amazon.in and healthrevolution.in.*

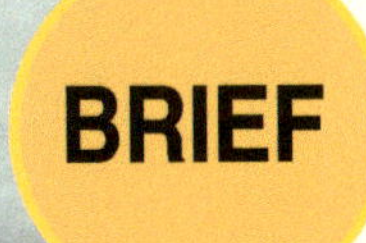

Preparation Time: **5 Min**
Soaking Time: **4-5 Hours or Overnight**
Cooking Time: **Not Required**
No. Of Servings: **3 Bowls**
Fridge Life: **3 Days**

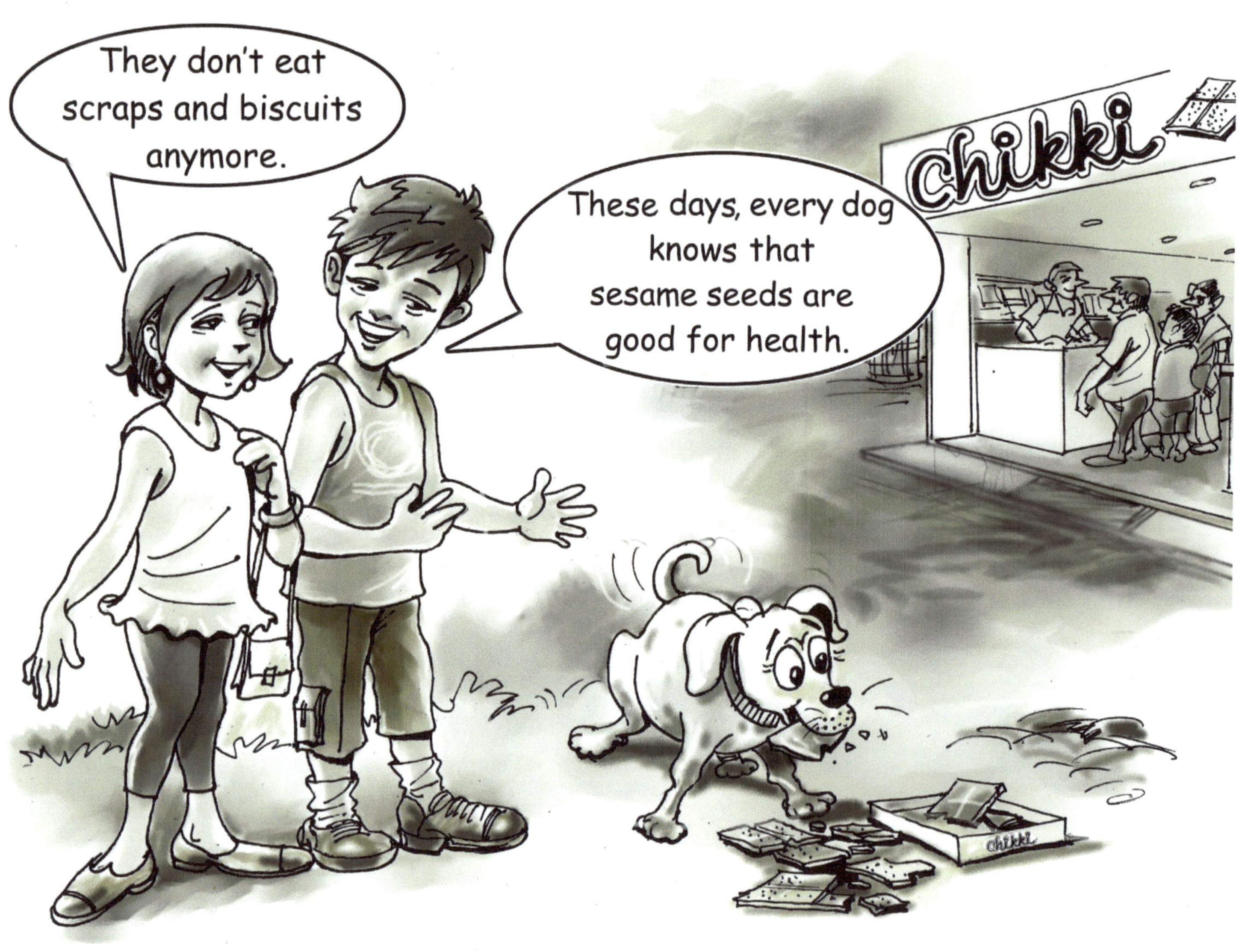
They don't eat scraps and biscuits anymore.
These days, every dog knows that sesame seeds are good for health.
Chikki
chikki

GENERAL REFERENCE GUIDE TO

CALCIUM IN FOODS

COH We has presented a general guide to the calcium values in our foods. We have chosen a more indigenous reference guide that we found easier to refer to, although there is no gold standard for reference across the world. We have done our best to put together the reference chart. Subsequently, you may find that the values are not absolute as there is no complete reference source for Indian foods. The charts also present other uses of the food and the various forms they may be consumed in your daily diet. Do note that the calcium values mentioned are in their raw form only, unless specified so. The calcium levels will change or reduce as you cook them (steam/ blanche/bake/microwave).

A. GREEN LEAFY VEGETABLES

A	Green Leafy Vegetables	Size of Serving	Calcium per serving	Calcium per 100gm or as stated	Always cooked/ Never Eat Raw	Smoothie & Salads	Cooking as bhaji	Chutny/ Dips	Savouries like muthia, Thepla	Cooked With Lentils	Soup
1	Phool Patta Gobi leaves	N A	N A	626mg	Both	Yes	Yes	Yes	Yes	Yes	No
2	Arvi leaves	1 cup (145g)	125mg	227mg	Cooked.	No	Yes	No	Patra	Yes	No
3	Methi sabji	1 Katori Cooked	395 mg	395 mg	Both	small quantity as it is bitter	Yes	No	Methi Vada	Besan	No
4	Shepu - Dill leaves (Anethum graveolens)	N A	N A	190mg	Both	Yes	Yes	Yes	Yes	With mung Daal	Yes
5	Dhania Patta/ Coriander Leaves	1/4 Cup (4 GM)	2.7 mg	184 mg	Both	Yes	Yes	Yes	Kothimbir Vadi	Yes	Lemon Coriander Soup
6	Mustard leaves or sai bhaji or sarsav bhaji	1 Cup Chopped (140mg) Cooked	104 mg	155 mg	Both	Yes	Yes	No	Yes	Yes	Yes
7	Bok Choy	N A	N A	105Mg	Both	Yes	Yes	No	Yes	Yes	Yes
8	Turnip greens	1 Cup Chopped (144 gm) Cooked	197 mg	710mg	Both	Yes	Yes	No	Yes	Yes	Yes
9	Fennel	N A	N A	109 mg	Both	Yes	yes	yes	Yes	No	Yes
10	Drumstick leaves (Moringa)	N A	N A	440 mg	Both	Yes	yes	No	Yes	Yes	Yes
11	Radish leaves	N A	N A	265 mg	Both	Yes	Yes	No	Yes	Yes	Yes
12	Rajgira(Amaranth) leaves	N A	N A	330 mg	Both	Yes	Yes	No	Yes	Yes	Yes
13	Beet greens	1 Cup (144gm) Cooked	164 mg	380 mg	Both	yes	No	No	Yes	Yes	Yes

A	Green Leafy Vegetables	Size of Serving	Calcium per serving	Calcium per 100gm or as stated	Always cooked/ Never Eat Raw	Smoothie & Salads	Cooking as bhaji	Chutny/ Dips	Savouries like muthia, Thepla	Cooked With Lentils	Soup
14	Curry leaves	N A	N A	810 mg	Both	yes	No	Yes	Yes	No	Yes
15	Chawli bhaji cow pea leaves	1 Cup(132g)	276 mg	372 mg	Both	yes	yes	No	Yes	Yes	Yes
16	Nagrvel or betal leaves	N A	N A	230 mg	Both	yes	No	No	No	No	No
17	Tamarind leaves Tender (Tamarindus indica)	N A	N A	101 mg	Both	young leaves	yes	yes, but mostly cooked like pachadi	Yes	Yes	Yes
18	Basil Leaves	2 tbsp chopped (5 gm)	9.3 mg	177 mg	Both	yes	Yes	yes. Pesto	Yes	No	Yes
19	Lettuce tree leaves Mature	N A	N A	320 mg	Both	yes	Yes	Yes	Yes	Yes	Yes
20	Mayalu Bhaji (Basella Alba), Malabar Spinach	N A	N A	200 mg	Both	yes	yes	No	Yes	Yes	Yes
21	Parsley	N A	N A	390 mg	Both	yes	yes	yes	Yes	Yes	Yes
22	Safflower leaves (Kusum Flowers)	N A	N A	185 mg	Both	young leaves	yes	No	yes	Yes	Yes
23	Mint leaves	N A	N A	200 mg	Both	yes	Yes	yes	Yes	No	Yes
24	Pumpkin Leaves	1 Cup (71 gm) Cooked	30.5 mg	392 mg	Both	young leaves	yes	yes	Yes	Yes	Yes
25	Kale	1 Cup Chopped (130 gm) Cooked	93.6 mg	150 mg	Both	yes	yes	yes	Yes	Yes	Yes
26	Collard Greens	1 Cup Chopped (190 gm) Cooked	266 mg	232mg	Both	yes	yes	yes	Yes	Yes	Yes
27	Agathi (Sesbania Grandiflora)	N A	N A	1130 mg	Both	Yes	Yes	Yes	Yes	Yes	Yes
28	Chana Leaves	N A	N A	340 Mg	Both	Yes	Yes	Yes	Yes	Yes	Yes
29	Bathua Leaves	1 Ounce (28 gm) cooked	97.7 mg	258 mg	Both	Yes	Yes	Yes	Yes	Yes	Yes
30	Carrot Leaves	N A	N A	340 Mg	Both	Yes	Yes	Yes	Yes	Yes	Yes
31	Broad bean leaves	N A	N A	111 Mg	Both	Yes	Yes	Yes	Yes	Yes	Yes
32	knol khol Ganth Gobi (kohlrabi) green leaves	N A	N A	368 mg	Both	Yes	Yes	No	Yes	Yes	Yes
33	Ponnanganni (Alternanthera sessilis) (Matsyakshi) Gudri sag	N A	N A	388 mg	Both	Yes	Yes	Yes	Yes	Yes	Yes
34	Leek	1 Leek 124 gm	37.2 mg	59 Mg	Both	Yes	Yes	Yes	Yes	Yes	Yes
35	Spinach	1 Katori	73 mg	99 mg	Both	Yes	Yes	Yes	Yes	Yes	Yes
36	Manathakkali (Solanum Nigrum)	N A	N A	410 Mg	Cooked	Yes	Yes	Yes	Yes	Yes	Yes
37	Celery leaves	N A	N A	230 mg	Both	Yes	Yes	Yes	Yes	Yes	Yes
38	Rape Leaves (Brassica napus)	N A	N A	370 mg	Both	Yes	Yes	No	Yes	Yes	Yes

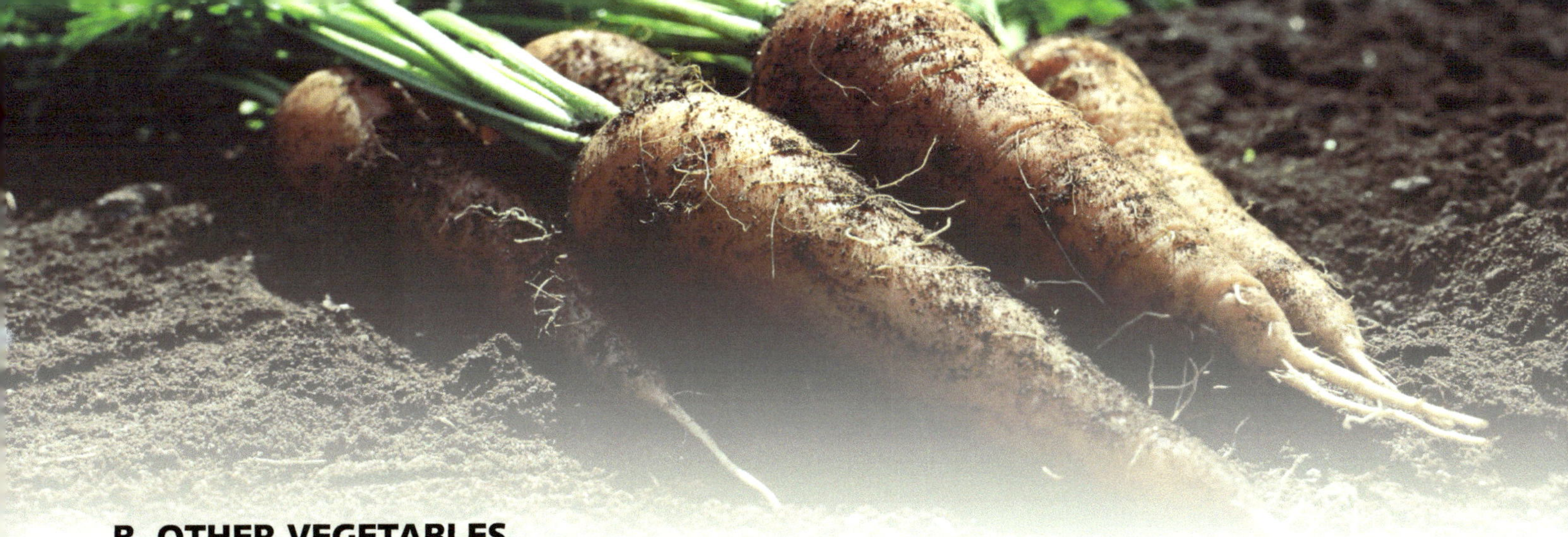

B. OTHER VEGETABLES

B	Other Vegetables	Size of Serving	Calcium per serving	Calcium per 100gm or as stated	Always cooked/ Never Eat Raw	Smoothie & Salads	Cooking as bhaji	Chutny/ Dips	Savouries like muthia, Patra, Thepla, pattice	Pancakes	Soup
1	Soyabean Sprouts	N A	N A	50 mg	Both	yes	yes	Yes	Yes	Yes	yes
2	Garlic	N A	N A	181 mg	Both	yes	yes	yes	Yes	Yes	Yes
3	Cabbage	1 Cup shredded (145 gm) cooked	43.5 mg	39 mg	Both	yes	Yes	Yes	Yes	Yes	yes
4	gawar or cluster beans	N A	N A	130 mg	Both	yes	yes	No	No	No	Yes
5	Lotus root	10 Slices cooked, 89 g	N A	405mg	Cooked	yes in salad, cooked.	yes	No	No	No	Yes
6	Sundakkai (Turkey Berry) Solanum torvum	N A	N A	390 mg	Cooked	No	Yes	Yes	No	No	yes
7	Pumpkin Flowers	1 Cup (134 gm)	49.6 mg	120 mg	Cooked	yes	yes	yes	yes	yes	yes
8	Sweet Potato	1 Cup (200 gm) cooked	76 mg	46 Mg	Cooked	No	yes	No	No	No	yes
9	butternut squash	1 Cup (205 gm) Cubes cooked	84 mg	48Mg	Cooked	No	Yes	No	No	No	Yes
10	carrot	1/2 Cup Slices cooked	23.4 mg	80 Mg	Both	yes	yes	Yes	Yes	Yes	Yes
11	Field beans (broad beans) Cooked	1 Cup (170 gm) cooked	61.2 mg	36 Mg	Can Eat raw	Yes	yes	No	No	No	yes
12	Bhindi	1/2 Cup slices (80 gm) cooked	61.6 mg	82 Mg	Both	No	Yes	No	No	No	yes
13	Broccoli	1/2 Cupchopped (78 gm) Cooked	31.2 mg	47 Mg	Both	Yes	Yes	Yes	Yes	Yes	Yes
14	Onions	1 ounce (28 mg) cooked	6.2 mg	47 Mg	Both	Yes	Yes	Yes	Yes	Yes	Yes

C. PULSES (AS FLOUR/ WET GROUNDED)

C	Pulses as Four/ Wet grinded	Size of Serving	Calcium per serving	Calcium per 100gm or as stated	Always cooked/ Never Eat Raw	Smoothie & Salads	Cooked with other veggies	Dips and Spreads	Savouries like muthia, Dhokla	Sprouts	Soup/ cooked lentils gravy
1	Black Turtle Beans	1 cup boiled	102 mg	160 mg	Yes	Yes	Yes	Yes	Yes	Yes	Yes
2	Chick peas / Chole	1 Cup (164 mg) cooked	80.4 mg	150 mg	Yes	Yes	Yes	Hummus	Yes	Yes	Yes
3	Kulthi (Horse Gram)	N A	N A	287 mg	Yes	Yes	Yes	Yes	Yes	Yes	Yes
4	White beans or Vaal	1 Cup (179 gm) cooked	161 mg	161 mg (1 cup cooked)	Yes	Yes	Yes	Yes	Yes	Yes	Yes
5	Rajma	1 Cup (177 gm) Cooked	49.6 mg	260mg	Yes	Yes	Yes	Yes	Yes	Yes	Yes
6	Desi chana/ Bengal Gram	N A	N A	202 mg	Yes	Yes	Yes	Yes	Yes	Yes	Yes
7	udad dal whole (Black gram)	1 Cup (172 gm) Cooked	46.4 mg	154 mg	Yes	Yes	Yes	Yes	Yes	no	Yes
8	Mung	1 Cup (125 gm) Cooked	55mg	124 mg	Yes	Yes	Yes	Yes	Yes	Yes	Yes
9	Soyabean	1 Cup (172 gm) Cooked	175 mg	240 mg	Yes	Yes	Yes	Yes	Yes	Yes	Yes
10	Kala Chana	1 Cup Cooked	80 mg	287 mg	Yes	Yes	Yes	Yes	Yes	Yes	Yes
11	Mung Daal Whole	N A	N A	75 mg	can eat raw but soaked in water for 2 hours	Yes	Yes	Yes	Yes	No	Yes
12	Mung Beans (Sprouted)	1 Cup Cooked (124 gm)	15 mg	14 mg	N A	Yes	Yes	Yes	Yes	No	Yes
13	Matki/ Moth beans/ Turkish Gram	N A	N A	202 mg	Yes	Yes	yes	Yes	Yes	Yes	Yes

D. GRAINS

D	Grains	Size of Serving	Calcium per serving	Calcium per 100gm or as stated	Always cooked/ Never Eat Raw	Roti, Rotla, breads	Pancakes	Porridge	Grain milk	Cooked With Lentils like Khichadi	Laddu
1	Oats	1 Cup (156 gm) Cooked	NA	84.3 mg	Always cooked	Yes	Yes	Yes	Yes	Yes	Yes
2	Ragi or finger millet	25 gm serving size, cooked	75 mg	364 mg	Always cooked	Yes	Yes	Yes	Yes	Yes	Yes
3	Bajra	N A	N A	42 Mg	Always cooked	Yes	Yes	Yes	Yes	Yes	Yes
4	Wheat	N A	N A	40.8 Mg	Always cooked	Yes	Yes	Yes	Yes	Yes	Yes
5	Quinoa	1 Cup Cooked (185 gm)	31.5 mg	47 mg	Always cooked	Yes	Yes	Yes	Yes	Yes	Yes

E. FRUITS

E	Fruits	Size of Serving	Calcium per serving	Calcium per 100gm or as stated	Raw	Smoothie & Salads	Cooking at times	Chutny/Dips	Ice cream		
	Dried Figs	5 whole figs	55 mg	(1/2 cup contains 120 mg)	Yes	yes	yes	Yes	yes		
1	Dried Apricot	1 ounce (28 gm)	40 mg	110 mg	Yes	yes	yes	yes	yes		
2	Black Currants	1 ounce (28 gm)	40 mg	130mg	Yes	Yes	yes	Yes	yes		
3	Blackberries	1 ounce (28 gm)	8.1 mg	(1 cup contains 40 mg)	Yes	yes	yes	Yes	yes		
4	Dried Dates	1 ounce (28 gm)	40 mg	120 mg	Yes	yes	yes	Yes	yes		
5	Orange	1 Orange	50 to 60 mg	N A	Yes	Yes	yes	Yes	yes		
6	Kiwi	1 Cup	60 mg	N A	Yes	Yes	yes	yes	yes		
7	Wood apple	1 ounce (28 gm)	40 mg	130 mg	Yes	yes	yes	Yes	yes		
8	Lime Peel	N A	N A	710 mg	Yes	Yes	yes	yes	yes		
9	Phalsa Grewia asiatica	N A	N A	129 mg	Yes	yes	yes	Yes	yes		
10	Sangri Khejri (Prosopis cineraria)	N A	N A	414 mg	No	No	yes	Yes	No		
11	Ker (Capparis decidua)	N A	N A	153 mg	No	No	yes	Yes	No		
12	Hingota (Balanites aegyptiaca)	N A	N A	147 mg	Yes	No	yes	Yes	No		
14	Mullberry	N A	N A	70 mg	yes	Yes	yes	No	Yes		
15	Prickly Pears	N A	N A	83.4 Mg	Yes	Yes	yes	No	Yes		

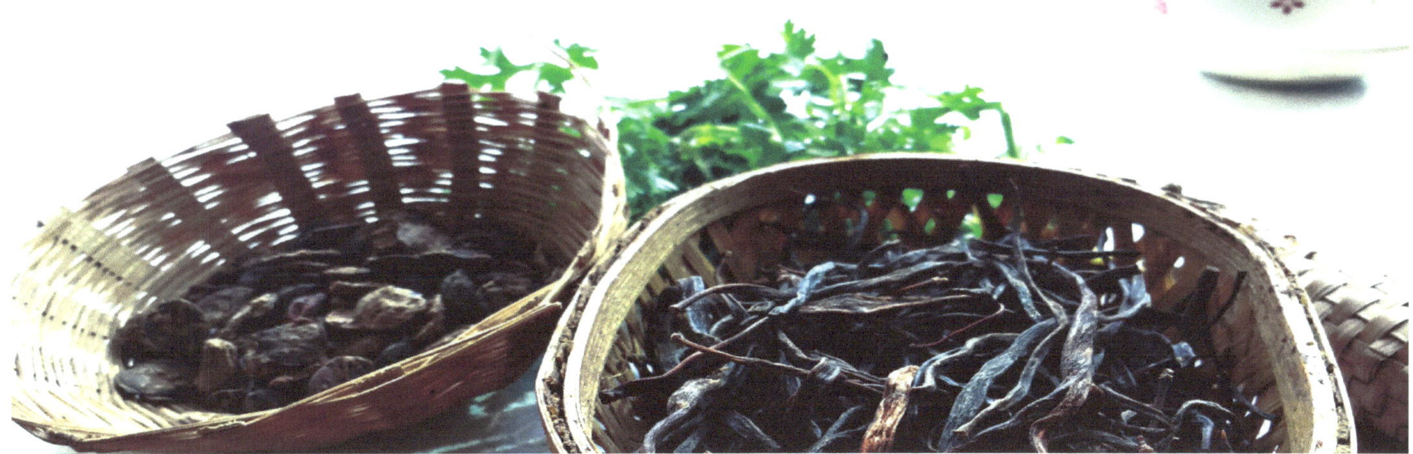

F. NUTS AND SEEDS

F	Nuts and Seeds	Size of Serving	Calcium per serving	Calcium per 100gm or as stated	Can Eat Raw	Dairy Free Milk	Butters/Dips	Sweets	Mukhvas	Other recipes
	calcium is well absorbed from seeds when they are ground.									
1	Sesame seeds	1 tbsp (25 gm)	363 mg	1283 mg	Yes	Yes	Butter, Tahini	Laddu, Gajak, chiki	Yes	Dips, Sweets, Chutneys , Oils
2	Almonds	Handful (25 gm)	58 mg	230 mg -260 mg	Yes	Yes	Butter, Cheese	Chiki, Choco balls	Yes	Dips, Sweets, Chutneys , Oils
3	Sun flower seeds	1 Cup(with hulls) Edible yeild 46 gm	35.9 mg	280 mg	Yes	Yes	Dip	No	Yes	Dips, Sweets, Chutneys , Oils
4	Amaranth/ Rajgira	1 Cup(246 gm)	116 mg	267 mg	No	Yes	Dip, Cheese	Chiki	No	Popps,Roti, poori, pancakes
5	Flaxseed	1 Cup Whole (168 gm)	428 mg	255 mg	Yes	No	Dip	Chiki	Yes	Sweets, Oils
6	Watermelon seeds kernel (Magajtari seeds)	1 Cup (108 gm)	58.3 mg	100 mg	Yes	Yes	Dip	Garnishing	Yes	Dips, Sweets, Chutneys , Oils
7	Mustard seeds	1 tbsp (11 gm)	57.3 mg	490 mg	Yes	No	Mustard Sauce	No	No	Dips, Chutneys , Oils
8	Charoli/Chironji (Buchanania lanzan)	N A	N A	279 mg	Yes	Yes	replacement of almonds		No	Can replace almonds
9	Safflower Seeds	1 Ounce(28 gm)	21.8 mg	78 mg	Yes	Yes	Dip	Garnishing	Yes	Nil
10	Pista	1 Cup (123 gm) Roasted	135 mg	107 mg	Yes	Yes	Dip, Cheese	Yes	Yes	Sweets
11	Walnut	1 Cup (117 gm)	115 mg	100mg	Yes	Yes	Dip, Cheese	Yes	Yes	Sweets, Smoothies, Oils
12	Chia seeds	1 Ounce(28 gm)	177 mg	631 mg	yes	No	No	Yes	No	Drinks, Smoothies
13	Basil or sabja seeds	N A	N A	177 mg	Yes	No	No	Yes	No	Drink
14	Buckwheat (Kutti no daro)	1 Cup (168 gm) Cooked	11.8 mg	114 mg	No	Yes	No	Pancakes	No	Roti
15	Poppy seeds	1 tbsp (9 gm)	126 mg	1372 mg	Yes	Yes	Gravy,Cheese	decoration	No	Sweets , Chutneys
16	Pine Nuts or Chilgoza	1 Cup (135 gm)	21.6 mg	16 mg	Yes	Yes	Pesto,Cheese	Yes	Yes	Sweets , Chutneys
17	Brazil Nuts	1 Cup Whole (133 gm)	213 mg	160 mg	Yes	Yes	Dip, Cheese	Yes	yes	Sweets , Chutneys

F	Nuts and Seeds	Size of Serving	Calcium per serving	Calcium per 100gm or as stated	Can Eat Raw	Dairy Free Milk	Butters/Dips	Sweets	Mukhvas	Other recipes
18	Hemp Seeds	100 gm	70 mg	70 mg	Yes	Yes	Dip,Cheese	No	Yes	Sweets , Chutneys
19	Water Lily Seeds	N A	N A	163 mg	Yes	No	No	Makhana Kheer	Yes	can eat roasted
20	Dry Coconut	N A	N A	400 mg	Yes	Yes	Dip	Yes	Yes	Sweets
21	Niger Seeds (Karale, Khurasni)	1 tbsp (15 gm)	40 mg	300mg	Yes	No	Dry Powder	No	No	Chutney, Powder
22	Kalonji or black onion seeds	N A	N A	1196 mg/1860 mg	Yes	No	No	decoration on nan	No	Chutney, Garnishing
23	Pumpkin Seeds	1 Cup (138mg)	59.3 mg	55 mg	Yes	Yes	Dip	Yes	Yes	Chuntey, Sweets
24	Fenugreek Seeds	1 tbsp(11 Gm)	19.4 mg	160 mg	After Soaking only	No	No	Yes	No	Raita

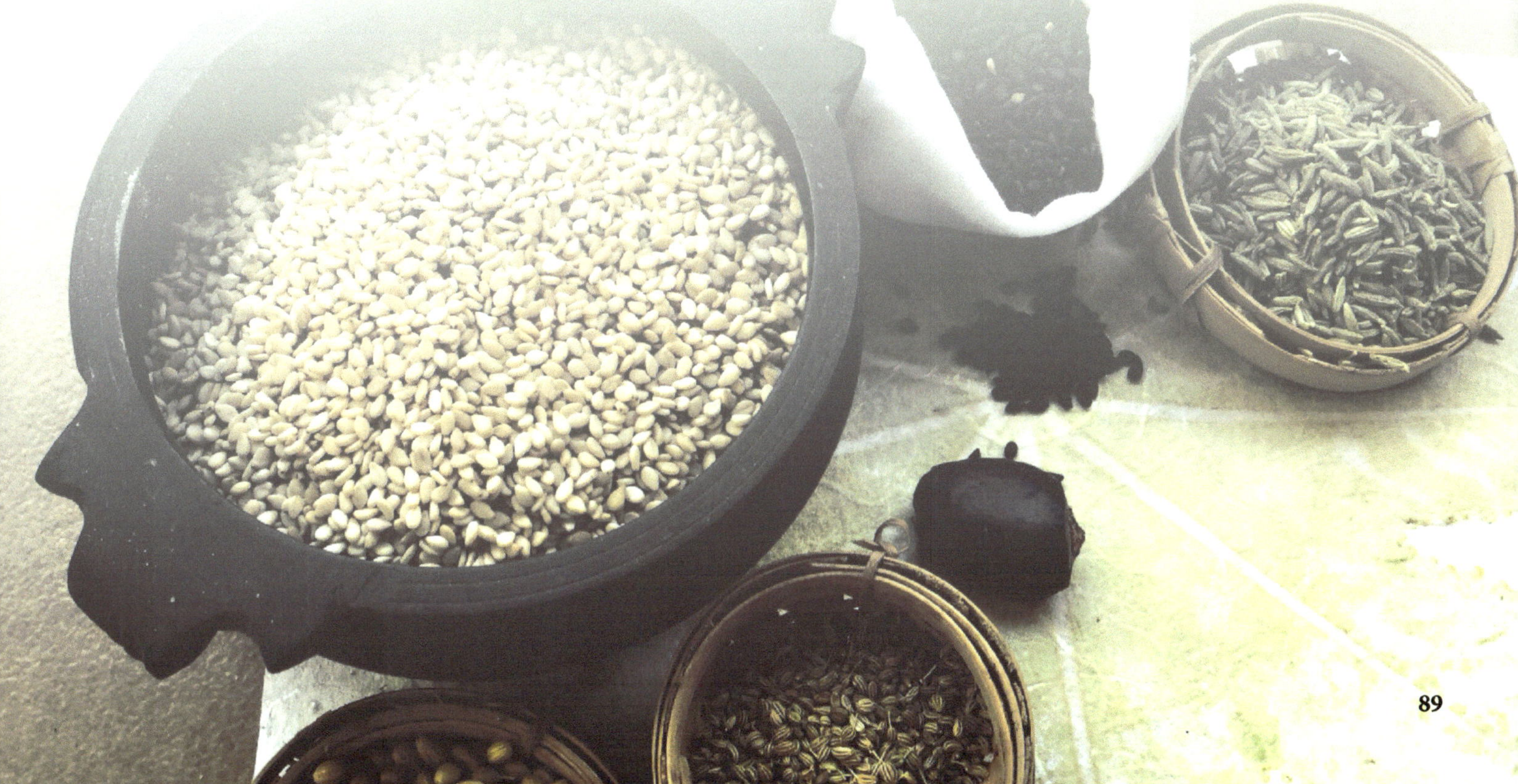

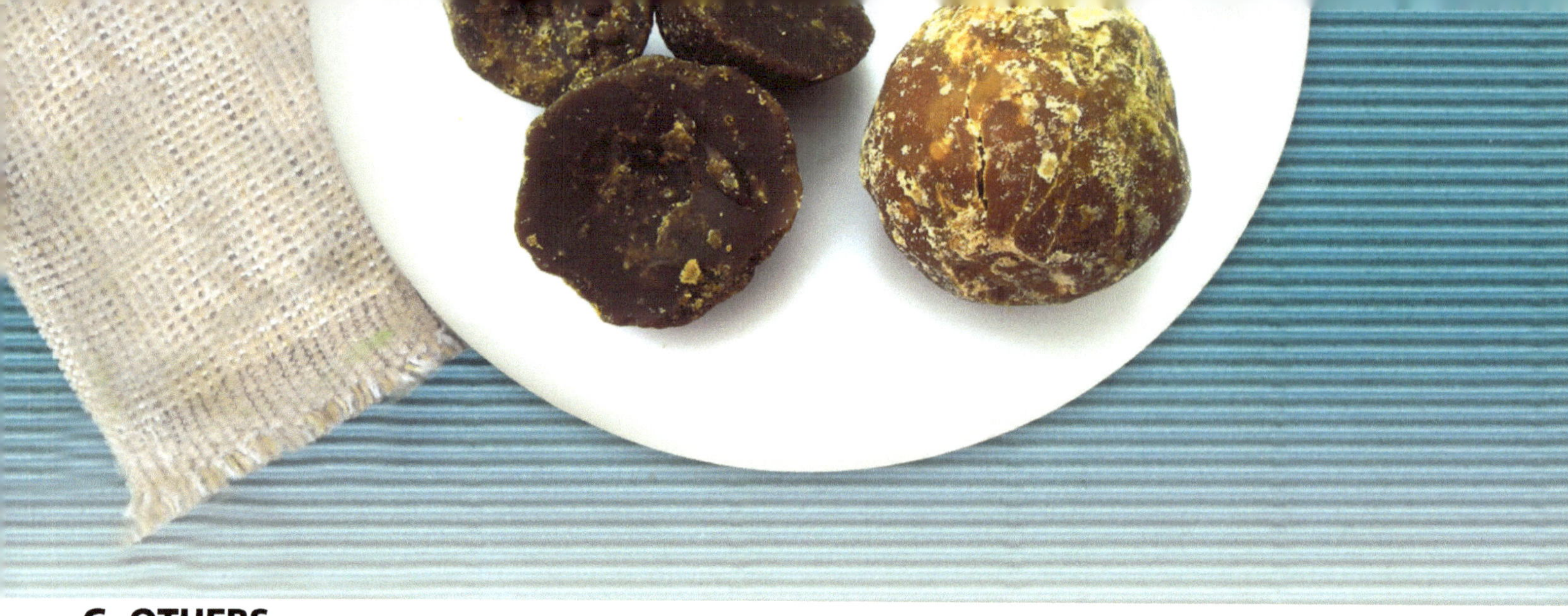

G. OTHERS

G	Other:	Calcium per 100gm or as stated	Use/s	Smoothie & Salads	Cooking as veggies	Chutny/ Dips	Savouries like muthia, Patra, Thepla	Cooked With Lentils	Soup
1	Black Strap Molasses	(1 tbsp. – 135 mg)	Natural Sweeteners	yes	NA	yes	yes	yes	yes
2	Jaggery (sago Palm)	1252mg	Natural Sweeteners	yes	NA	yes	yes	yes	yes
3	Jaggery Date Palm	363 mg	Natural Sweeteners	yes	NA	yes	yes	yes	yes
4	Jaggery Coconut Palm	1638 mg	Natural Sweeteners	yes	NA	yes	yes	yes	yes
5	Jaggery (Fan Palm)	225 mg	Natural Sweeteners	yes	NA	yes	yes	yes	yes
6	Cane Jaggery	80 Mg	Natural Sweeteners	yes	NA	yes	yes	yes	yes
6	kakvi	80 Mg	Natural Sweeteners	yes	NA	yes	yes	yes	yes
7	soya tofu	350 mg	Cooked Only	yes	Scrambled	yes	yes	yes	yes
8	Nori Rolls	280 Mg	Sushi rolls	yes	NA	NA	yes	yes	yes
9	Methi Sprouts	176 Mg	Salads	yes	Yes	NA	yes	yes	yes
10	Wheat Grass	429Mg	Salad/ Juice	yes	Yes	NA	yes	yes	yes
11	Barley Grass	775 Mg	Salad / Jiuce	yes	Yes	NA	yes	yes	yes

H. MAJOR SPICES

H	Major Spices	Calcium per 100gm or as stated	Raw	Sprouts
1	Celery seeds 100gm 1767 mg calcium ajwain or ajmo	1034 mg	Yes	NA
2	Mustard Seeds	490 mg	Yes	Yes
3	Fenugreek Seeds	160 mg	Yes	Yes
4	Coriander Seeds	630mg	Yes	Yes
5	Asafoetida	690 mg	No	No
6	Cardamom	130 mg	Yes	No
7	Dry chillies	160 mg	Yes	No
8	Dry cloves	740 mg	Yes	No
9	Cumin Seeds	1080 mg	Yes	No
10	Mango Powder	180 mg	Yes	No
11	Dry black pepper	460 mg	Yes	No
12	Turmeric	150 mg	Yes	No
13	Green Pepper	270mg	Yes	No
14	Cinnamon	1002 mg	Yes	No
15	Tamarind pulp	170mg	Yes	No
16	Garden Cress Seeds(Lepidium Sativum) Halim, Chandrashoor, Asalu	377 mg	No	yes
17	Indian Long Pepper - Pippali	1230 mg	No	No

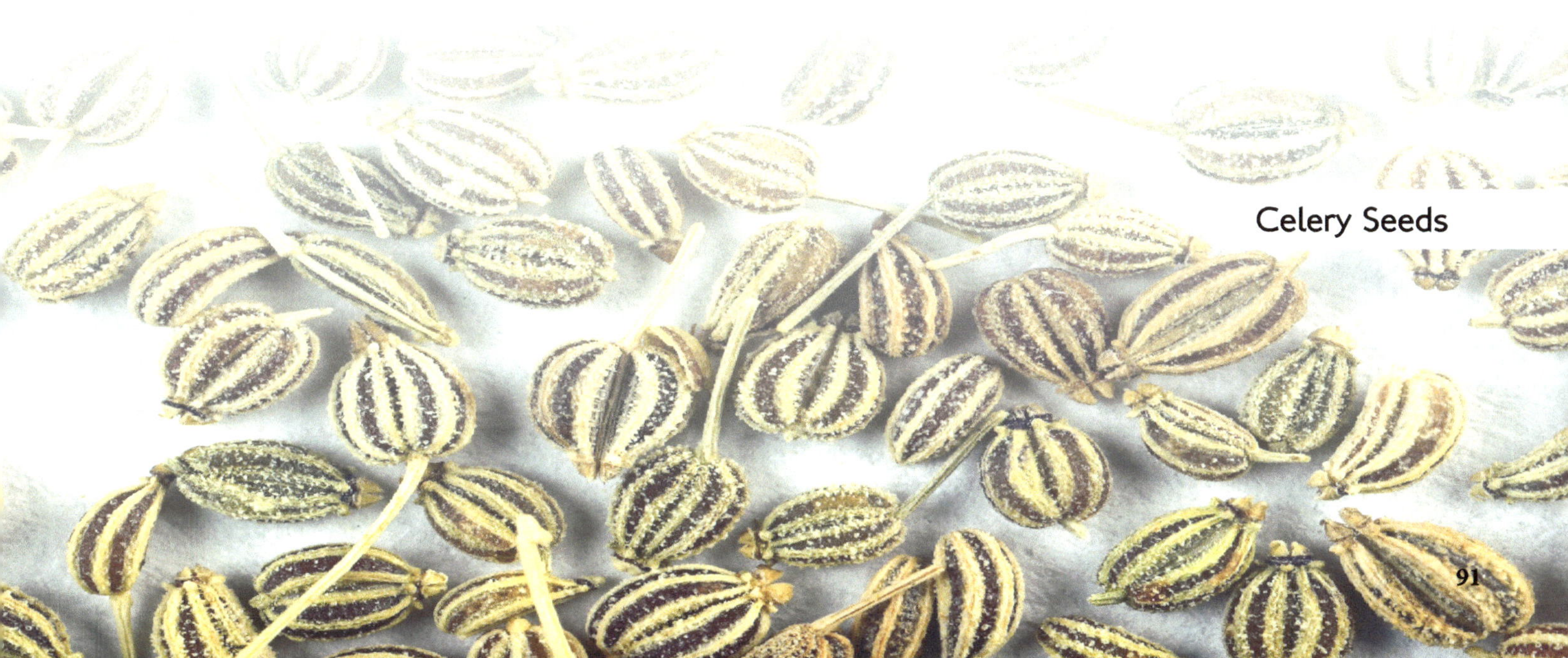
Celery Seeds

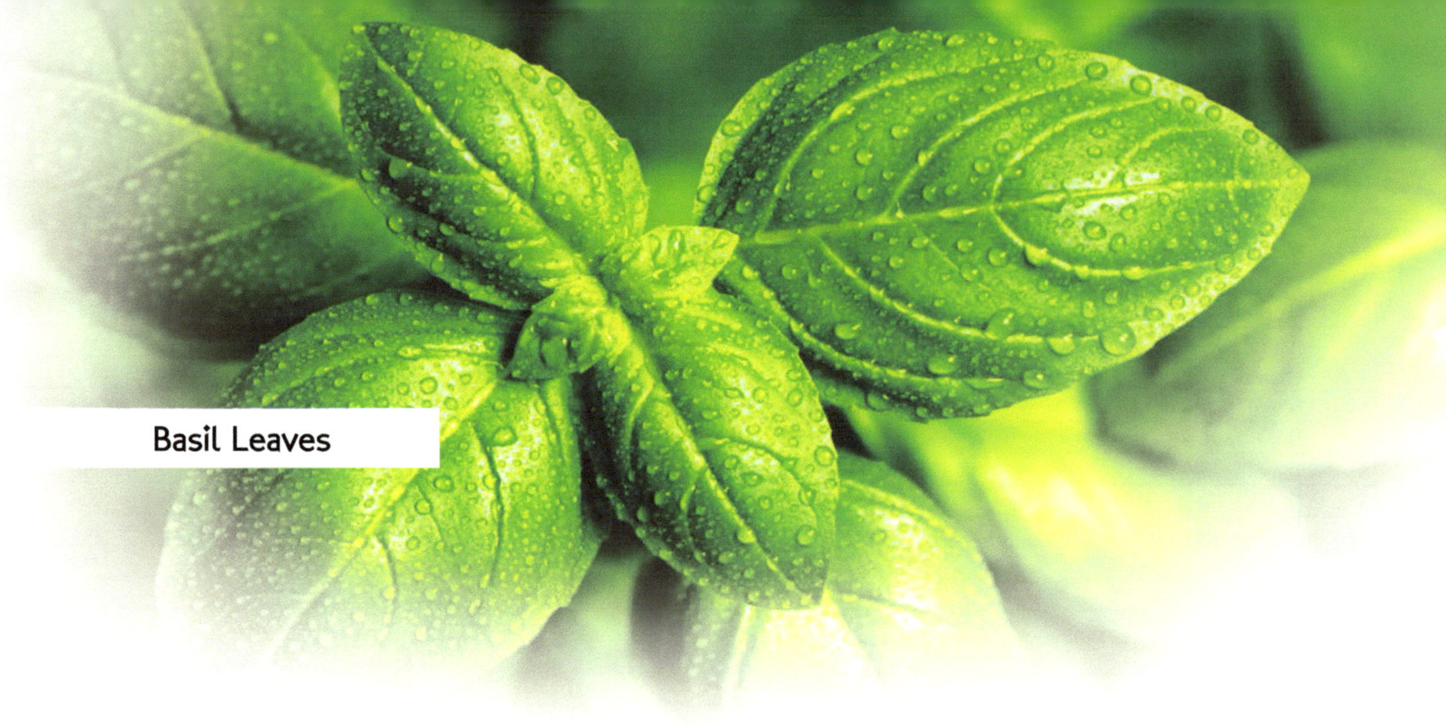

I. ALL DRIED HERBS

(Used in cooking to enhance flavour of foods)

I	All dried herbs	Used in cooking to enhance flavour of foods.		Calcium per 100gm or as stated
1	Basil(100gm)			2240Mg
2	Marjoram			1990Mg
3	Thyme			1890 Mg
4	Dill			1780Mg
5	Oregano			1580 Mg
6	Parsley			1080Mg

Ref: 1. Nutritive Value of Indian Foods by Gopalan, BV Rama Sastri and BS Balasubramanium
2. http://www.medindia.net

"Only plant sources of calcium should be eaten because this natural calcium has a genetic code to be deposited into the bones to make them healthy."

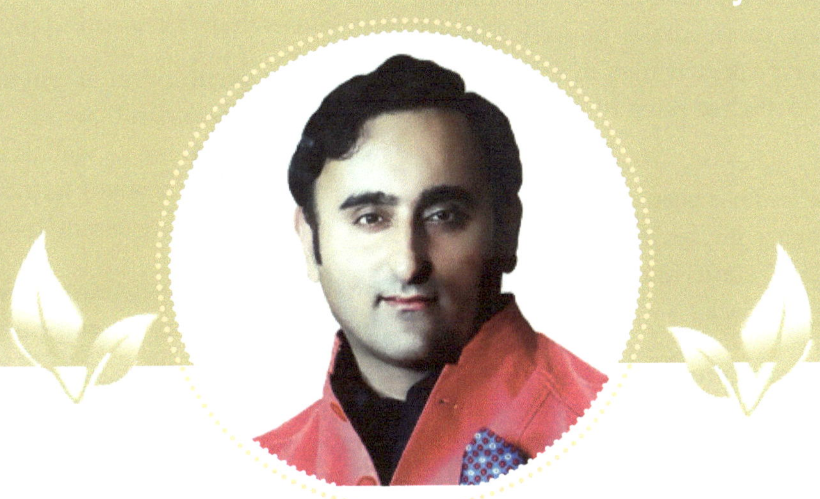

Dr Paawan Wadhawan on Calcium

Dr Paawan Wadhawan MBBS, MD (Internal Medicine) is a Consultant Physician, Diabetologist and Nutritionist. Through the years he has successfully reversed diabetes, hypertension and heart diseases of his patients with the power of natural foods. His simple methods have brought about a revolution in the field of nutrition. He endeavours to provide his patients with the best tested research work towards living a positive life, and they are often encouraged by his positive spirit. He has simplified many medical concepts for better understanding and his aim is to create awareness of the power of plant-based foods.

Can a diet, be it plant-based or vegan or raw or any other help to reverse bone loss/ improve bone health?

Whole and plant based foods, and sufficient exposure to the sun is in fact the only way to improve mineralization of bones and hence reverse bone loss (improved bone health).

Can a diet improve bone health?

It usually takes about 1 week to improve the symptoms of osteoporosis when a patient shifts to whole food and plant-based diet, provided his Vitamin D status is not deficient. (Note: Symptoms will vary on a case-to-case basis). Dexa scans can demonstrate an improvement in bone densities by 3 months.

Are there any age limitations beyond which there cannot be bone improvement?

Usually bone disease in old age depends upon what was the peak bone density during adolescence. Peak bone mass is inversely proportional to the amount of milk intake during the childhood i.e. more intake of milk during childhood leads to lower peak densities in adolescence which ultimately leads to higher rates of fractures and osteoporosis in old age.

But still, it is possible and has been demonstrated that bone density in old age starts improving once the patient improves his/her Vitamin D status and shifts exclusively to whole food and plant-based diet.

What aspect of calcium consumption is the most misunderstood by people?

Milk is the only source of calcium. This is the most common myth which prevails among Indian people. But it has been proved in many studies published in International Medical Journals that galactose present in milk is responsible for senescence and early death of osteoblasts 'the bone forming cells', which leads to demineralization of bones and hence osteoporosis.

Also people think that calcium supplementation is compulsory once we start aging.

But the scientific data is totally contradictory to this belief. Calcium is more readily absorbable from greens such as kale and broccoli than dairy milk. Getting your calcium from plants also means that getting fibre, antioxidants, and foliates as well, whereas dairy calcium comes with saturated fat, hormones, and cholesterol.

Calcium supplements are not recommended as they might increase your risk of other conditions like coronary artery disease, stroke and fatal heart attack. Omnivores, raw food enthusiasts, and vegans alike all are found to be eating calcium deficient diets. Long-time vegans appear to have the same bone mineral density as omnivores of a similar height, weight, and activity level, despite the fact that they may only consume about half the amount of calcium as their dairy-eating counterparts.

High consumption of phytates and fibre appears to enhance bone-mineral density. Moreover, fortified soy milk is absorbed just as well as cow's milk by osteopenic post-menopausal women (although you must shake the soy milk carton to distribute the calcium).

What can be the one statement to help us clear the fog about calcium consumption?

Only natural or plant sources of calcium should be eaten because this natural calcium has enzymatic activity i.e. it has a life and genetic code to be deposited into the bones to make them healthy.

The calcium consumed from milk and calcium tablets are dead calcium sources, hence no genetic programming about its target or where the elements consumed have to go. Consequently, the elements will be assimilated in the body and be deposited at the wrong places, like the gall bladder and kidneys, forming stones or be deposited in coronaries of the heart or the carotid arteries, leading to heart attack or stroke and so on.

Do women require more calcium as compared to men,
especially post-menopause?

Post-menopausal requirements of women are a little more than men due to fall in there estrogen levels, which helps in maintaining the bone mineral density. But this extra need can be easily fulfilled by eating calcium-rich plants like moringa, spinach, almonds, fig and oranges.

Is calcium related to weight gain or weight loss?

No clear cut data is available on relationship of weight and calcium intake. Some supplement companies advertise that weight loss is associated with calcium supplements, but that cannot be relied upon.

Can you elaborate on importance of minerals for bone health.

Calcium can only be absorbed from the gut if diet is not deficient in magnesium, phosphorus and zinc, and the Vitamin D Levels of the body are adequate. These trace minerals are available only in natural plant-based sources of calcium and not in calcium tablets.

At what age should one take the first Bone Density test and Serum Calcium test? And at what frequency should one take re-tests after the first base-line test?

It has been proved now in International Medical studies that routine annual check-ups are a total waste of money. So it is advisable to go for bone testing if you have symptoms of osteoporosis or suffering from recurrent fractures. But this holds true only if you are on WFPB diet. If you are not following the whole food plant-based diet, then better to go for a bone check-up immediately after menopause and then repeat it annually.

Suggest a 7-day Meal plan to for those who are just starting on wfpd?

For a 7-day Plan to Boost Bone & Teeth, eat the following:

- Whole & plant-based food diet (strictly)
- 2 servings of steamed green leaves 50gm each
- Moringa and spinach
- 5 water-soaked almonds, daily
- Small piece of fig, daily
- Oranges
- Prunes, plums & peaches, if available

NOTE: Take half hour sunlight in between 11am to 2pm specially in summer, or take water soluble Vitamin D supplements 2000 IU daily

- Take 250mcg of Vit B12 daily in the form of cyanocobalamin
- Walk for 1 hour daily
- Rinse your teeth after every meal

REFERENCES

1. *Burckhardt, P. (2016). The role of low acid load in vegetarian diet on bone health: a narrative review.*

   Swiss Medical Weekly.

2. *Michaelsson K, Wolk A, Langenskiold S, Basu S, Warensjo Lemming E, Melhus H et al.*

   Milk intake and risk of mortality and fractures in women and men: cohort studies. BMJ. 2014;349(oct27 1):g6015-g6015.

3. *[Internet]. 2017 [cited 30 November 2017]. Available from: https://www.hopkinsmedicine.org/news/media/releases/calcium_supplements_may_damage_the_heart*

4. *Bloomfield HE, Wilt TJ. Evidence Brief: Role of the Annual Comprehensive Physical Examination in the Asymptomatic Adult. 2011 Oct. In: VA Evidence-based Synthesis Program Evidence Briefs [Internet]. Washington (DC):* Department of Veterans Affairs (US); 2011

Final Notes

Ayurveda With Plant-Based Lifestyle

In India, we apply knowledge of Ayurveda while eating foods. Ayurveda takes into account the essential nature of food and the constitution of the person eating food along with the season and place where one stays. It is possible that you can digest one food better than other, or you could be hypersensitive to some foods. Some foods increase your pitta, while some may increase your vata, causing imbalance of tridosha as per ayurvedic principles. Try to find out which foods suits you and which foods don't, and do apply some additional wisdom and consume foods as per your own constitution.

Pregnancy & Breast-Feeding Stages

A pregnant woman's need for calcium goes up in the third trimester, when the baby's skeleton is rapidly developing. The fetal skeleton is genetically coded to get what it needs, even if it has to leach essentials from its mother's bones. Also, a woman's body can sense the increased needs of the fetus and produce more vitamin D. This enables pregnant women and nursing mothers to absorb more of the calcium that's in their food. NOTE: Newborns to 11 months old require anywhere from 200-260mg of calcium a day. The only type of milk babies should have is breast milk.

Bioavailability & Unavailability

Bioavailability is the key to calcium assimilation in the body or the degree to which a nutrient is utilized and how well the calcium absorbed and incorporated into our bones. Vitamin D synergizes calcium absorption in the blood. On the other hand, some greens that are high in oxalates (oxalic acid) are also called antinutrients. The oxalates are naturally occurring compounds that bind to the calcium, making some of it unavailable to your body. Some foods that inhibit absorption of calcium are spinach and rhubarb.

Calcium Super Foods

Many of the foods suggested in the section are locally available. Here is a list of calcium superfoods that are bioavailable as well:

1. **Sesame Seeds (Black & White):** Both types of sesame seeds are superfoods for the body. They are rich with many nutrients and must be included in your diet.
2. Nachani (Finger Millets or Ragi): Introduced in one of our first recipes in the book, they make a nutritious meal or snack.
3. **Turnip Greens, Moringa & Curry Leaves**: High levels of nutrients in these leaves can enhance health and help prevent disease.
4. **Sprouts**: One of our favourite foods, sprouts (all types) offer a lot of flexibility–they can be used in chats, salads or eaten as mono-meals. Eat them as often as possible.
5. **Carom Seeds (Bishop Weeds) (Ajwain/ Ajmo)**: This spice is loaded with calcium and has a range of medicinal properties. Make sure to include this tiny powerhouse in your diet.
6. **Broccoli, Kale & Bok Choy**: These veggies are now on top of our list of superfoods and grown in India. They may not be easily found in all markets, but try to access it, when possible.
7. **Soy family**: Tofu or soy milk–both are best consumed when home-made, else check the labels and make sure the soybeans are organic or GMO-free. Some soy types will be fortified with calcium, while others may have less calcium–both help protect bones against osteoporosis. Edemame are soybeans that are harvested before they mature are now cultivated in India, and are excellent calcium resources. They can be lightly steamed and consumed. NOTE: Eat processed soy foods in moderation.
8. **Knol Khol (Kolrabi) Greens**: Also known as German turnip, the greens are abundant in carotenes, vitamins A, K, minerals, and the B-complex group.
9. **Fresh Fruits**: Along with this food, do consume as much Vitamin C as possible. Try to have 2 servings a day, when possible as they help assimilate the complex proteins and calcium much better.
10. **Bright Whole Foods**: Consume as much of bright coloured fruits and veggies with calcium foods as possible for maximum all-round benefits.

Information Gaps

It can be observed from the dietary recommendation guidelines presented by organizations in US, UK and India that they have no common baseline, as they do not agree with the calcium levels we require.

At a seminar at the Royal Society Of Medicine in London for the event 'Starving For Truth: Nutrition Myths And Controversies' on 6 November 2017, Prof. Susan Fairweather- Tait throws light on the gaps in knowledge surrounding calcium intake requirements.

Along the same lines, the British Medical Journal (BMJ) has stated in one of its papers that clear guidance on calcium and vitamin D supplements is lacking. It can be very confusing for you to understand how much calcium or vit D3 you require at any stage of your life. The recommendations for daily calcium intake vary by country. So how much calcium to we need? And which guidelines should you follow?

Recommendations

Although there are no common guidelines to indicate how much is less or how much is more, the best practice is to eat in balance and ensure that your calcium dietary intake does not fall below 600-800mg a day. If you have osteoporosis or are at risk of having it, then sim for the US guidelines and follow the **10- Step Program on Pg102.**

TIP: Do not avoid oxalate or phytate-containing foods. Such foods have other nutrients that are also very good for our bodies. Boil high-oxalate foods for better calcium consumption. Also, when it comes to phytates in foods like seeds, nuts and grains, you can sprout them to get improved mineral nourishment. Remember to eat all foods in rotation.

Calcium dietary Recommendation Comparison Between 3 Countries

		American Bone Health	British Dietetic Ass.	Nutrition Foundation of India
No	**Group Age (years) / Calcium (mg) per day**	**US**	**UK**	**Recommended By ICMR Group, 2009**
1	Children 1-3	700	350	600
2	Children 4-8	1000	450	600
3	Children 7-10	NA	550	Yrs. 1-9 = 600
4	Ages 10-12	1300	NA	Boys:600 / Girls:700
5	Children 9-18	1300	NA	(Age grps further broken)
6	Ages 13-15	1300	800 (girls)/ 1000 (boys)	Boys:800 / Girls:700
5	Adolescents 11-18	1300	-	NA
6	Ages 16-18	1300	-	Boys:600/ Girls:600
6	Ages 19-50	1000	700	600
7	Ages (Pregnant or Nursing)	1300	NA	NA
8	Ages (Pregnant or Nursing)	1000	1250	1200
10	Men: 51-70	1000	> 55 Yrs. 1200	600
11	Women: 51-71	1200	NA	600
9	Women past menopause	NA	1200	600
10	Ages 71+	1200	1200	600
11	Osteoporosis Adults	NA	1000	NA

Ref Links *(1) American Bone health: (https://americanbonehealth.org/ nutrition/ how-much-calcium-and-vitamin-d-do-you-need/)*
(2)BDA: https://www.bda.uk.com/foodfacts/Calcium.pdf
(3) Nutrition Foundation of India: http://www. nutritionfoundationofindia.org/pdfs/ BulletinArticle/Pages_from_final_ Bulletin_January_2010_1.pdf

What About My
Vitamin D3?

Vitamin D is a fat-soluble vitamin (actually a hormone) that is responsible for increasing intestinal absorption of calcium, magnesium, and phosphate among other elements. There are two forms of vitamin D: Vitamin D2 or ergocalciferol, is commonly found in foods, and vitamin D3 or cholecalciferol is made by the body naturally when skin is exposed to the sun.

Sunlight is a natural source of vitamin D3, and people who spend a lot of time working in offices or patients who stay indoors are most likely to be deficient in it.

Some studies suggest that the time of day when you receive sunlight affects how well your body absorbs vitamin D3. Cholecalciferol is made in the skin following UVB light exposure. It is converted in the liver to calcifediol (25-hydroxyvitamin D) which is then converted in the kidney to calcitriol (1,25-dihydroxyvitamin D). One of its actions is to increase the uptake of calcium by the intestines. Calcitriol then prompts the body to produce a handful of proteins in the gut whose job it is to transport calcium from the inside area of the intestine, through its wall, and into the blood.

Are D3 Supplements Ineffective?

Although some experts advocate that that the best form of vitamin D supplement to take is vitamin D3, recent studies by Dr Mark J Bolland, associate professor at the University of Auckland in New Zealand published in the Lancet Diabetes & Endocrinology prove otherwise. In a CNN Health feature, the team indicated that Vitamin D does not prevent fractures or falls, or have a meaningful effect on bone mineral density, concluding that there is little justification in taking them to 'maintain or improve musculoskeletal health'.

In another study by Dr Clifford Rosen, professor of medicine at the Tufts University School of Medicine and Senior Scientist at Maine Medical Center, told CNN that it's generally better to get vitamin D from the sun and food than from supplements. This way, D3 is more natural and easier for the body to absorb.

What To Do:

- While many experts advise people to avoid sunlight between the hours of 10am and 2pm or 3pm to help protect their skin from cancer, data shows the body actually absorbs vitamin D3 better during this time.
- Although there is no clear information about how much D3 we require, most medical experts agree that people need to expose their arms and legs to the sun's rays for between five and 30 minutes twice a week—though this amount is likely higher for people with darker skin as melanin blocks some of the rays. So we cannot emphasize enough about the importance of walking outdoors as often as you can.

STEPS for better bone health

Weak bones may seem unavoidable and a symptom of aging, but there is a lot we can do at any stage in life to make sure bones improve and stay healthy.

1 Stop Consuming Dairy, Meat & Eggs

The first step is to eliminate dairy, meat and eggs. Research has established that animal proteins are the cause of a host of health issues including osteoporosis and inhibits optimum assimilation of calcium in the body. Switch to a whole and plant based food lifestyle. There are plenty of delicious recipes in this book and other vegan reference books out there that can guide you through the process

2 Know Your Family History

Family history is the key indicator of bone health and many health conditions. If your grandparent, parent or sibling has or has had osteoporosis, you are more likely to develop it. Ask your parent and grandparents about their health history, if you have not yet done so. Make a note of it and start taking corrective measures as early as possible.

3 Boost Calcium Consumption

The body understands consumption of natural foods better than factory-made tablets. The body will instantly take to calcium-rich foods like broccoli, mustard leaves, curry leaves and other foods mentioned throughout this book. Calcium is essential for proper muscle functioning, nerve signaling, hormone secretion, and blood pressure

4 Partner With Vitamin D

Walk regularly outdoors during the daytime for about at least half an hour. Vitamin D's importance to bone health has been proven in studies. Also, the skin at a later stage can lose its ability to create Vitamin D from the sun. So start walking in the mornings or mid-mornings as often as you can.

5 Join Hands with Vitamins B 12

Check your B12 level annually if normal, and then check it once every 2 years. Dr Tushar Mehta, Family & Emergency Medicine, Canada, advises, "Take supplements of about 2,000mcg every week OR 1,000 mcg once or twice a week OR 10-20mcg once a day. NOTE: B12 shots are not required unless there are special medical conditions."

6 Other Vitamins & Minerals

Other minerals like potassium, magnesium and phosphorus and Vitamins like C and K are known to boost calcium absorption and boost bone health. Eat a lot of bright coloured fruits like oranges and apples and veggies like red peppers and purple cabbages. Also eat raw vegetables and sesame seeds. Include lots of sprouts and lentils, and consume a handful of dry fruits, nuts and seeds regularly.

7 Prioritize Exercising

Regular exercise is essential to keep a number of health issues at bay, and bone health is no exception. In fact, living a sedentary lifestyle is considered a risk factor for osteoporosis. Yoga, walking, jumping rope and climbing stairs keep bones the strongest. These exercises help improve your strength and balance and helps prevent falls–and the associated fractures–in those who already have osteoporosis.

8 Cut The Caffeine

Studies have shown that caffeine is not good for the bones. Caffeine consumption can interfere with the body's ability to absorb calcium. One study showed that drinking more than two cups of coffee per day accelerated bone loss in subjects who also didn't consume enough calcium. In another study, more than 18 ounces of coffee per day can accelerate bone loss by negatively interacting with vitamin D. So enjoy the latte or java, but keep it in moderation, but boost the calcium-rich natural foods in your regular diet as well.

9 Cut Down Alcohol, Tobacco & Smoking

Although heavy drinking will take a toll on overall health in the long run, and can cause bone loss (because it interferes with vitamin D doing its job), moderate consumption i.e. one drink per day for women, two per day for men is fine. On the other hand, multiple studies have shown that smoking and tobacco consumption decreases bone mass and can prevent the body from efficiently absorbing calcium.

10 Balance Your Diet

The recipes shown in the book present broad guidelines to enable you to choose your foods better. Eat the suggested foods in moderation and broaden the range of foods rich with essential nutrients. Remember to include all forms of lentils and beans in your diet as well. Do not repeat recipes too often. Eat fresh, local, organic and seasonal foods.

About Dr Rupa Shah

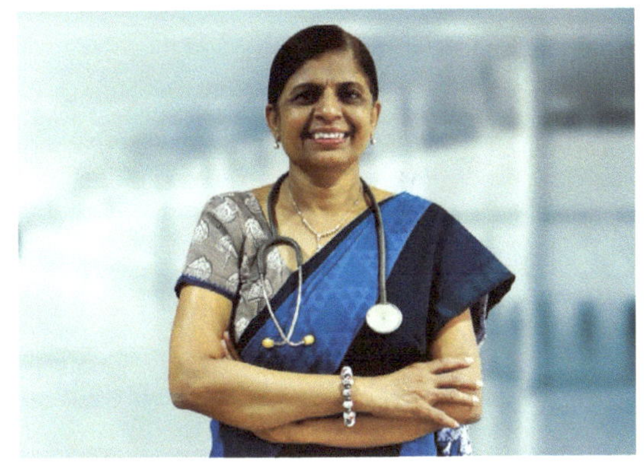

Dr Rupa A Shah is the Founder and Director of Health Revolution India that has been established in December 2014. She is an MBBS based in Mumbai and has been healing patients for the past 40+ years. She has also studied 'Lifestyle Medicine' from the Harvard Medical School, Boston, USA.

She is the winner of JITO 2018 award for exceptional contribution towards ahimsa. Dr Shah has published her maiden book project 'Dairy Alternatives' in 2015, and on popular demand, she translated the book in Gujarati and Hindi as well. The book has been amongst the top 3 Amazon bestsellers and still continues to be in popular demand. Additionally, she is co-founder of The Ahimsa Parmo Dharma in 2016. She helped organize many vegan festivals in India. One of them is known as One Earth Festival, it is India's largest vegan festival that aims to spread the message of ahimsa or compassion.

As a doctor, Dr Rupa Shah has dedicated her life to researching bio-energy and flower remedies and is sharing her findings with practitioners all over the world. She uses her allopathic knowledge in her research to present it scientifically amongst her colleagues. As an Allopathic physician, her comprehensive training has enabled her to persuade her peers and colleagues to consider using Bio- Energy Remedies successfully. Finally, she helps people become healthy by reversing lifestyle related diseases like diabetes, hypertension, obesity, high cholesterol, thyroid through plant-based food and lifestyle modification.

She has been invited as a guest speaker to various organizations in Mumbai and across India. She has delivered lectures at various seminars like the International Flower Remedies Essences Conference in Australia, Canada, U.K., USA, Germany, Italy, France, Spain, Switzerland, Brazil, Greece, Portugal, Ireland, Turkey, Dubai and India.

Other Publications by Dr Rupa Shah

ORDER YOUR COPY NOW

for Rs. **150 only**

www.healthrevolution.in

Also available on amazon.in

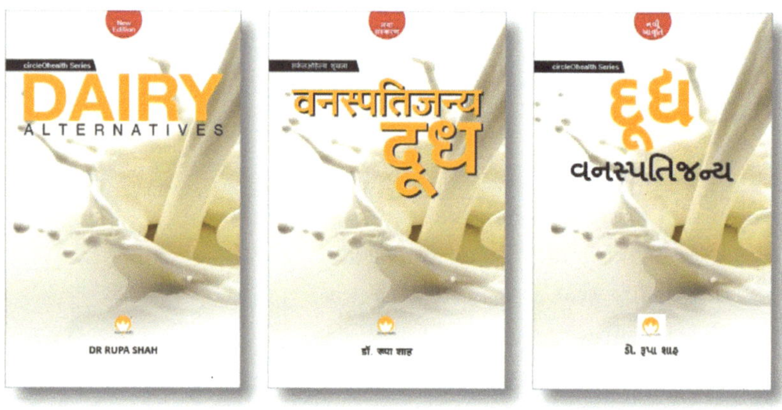

This handbook (available in 3 languages) of over 30 delectable dairy-free recipes is the ultimate guide for those just starting on their vegan or plant-based journey. Plus a special section on dairy-free curds, butters and ice-cream! This book is more than just a recipe book. It is loaded with handy tips to perk up your foods and lifestyle and also includes a Kitchen Transformation chart.

Paperback: 52 pages
Dimensions: 5.25″ x 8.50″
Publisher: CircleOHealth
Language: English, Hindi & Gujrati